REAL-WORLD CHALLENGES IN CLINICAL MEDICINE

PRACTICAL CLINICAL SCENARIOS TO STRENGTHEN DECISION-MAKING SKILLS

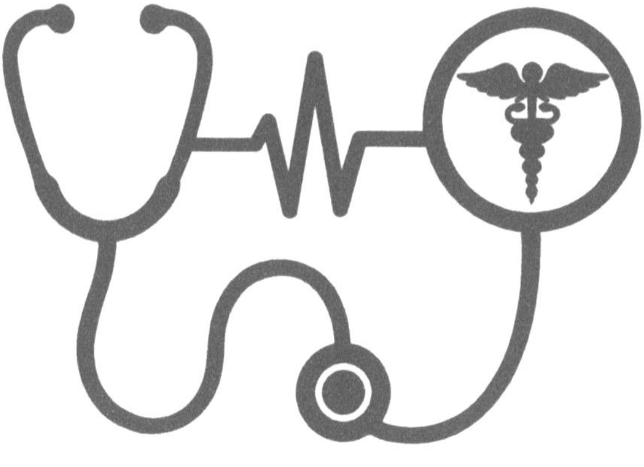

DR OMAR HASSOUNA

BROWN DOG BOOKS

First published 2026

Published under licence by Brown Dog Books and
The Self-Publishing Partnership Ltd, 10b Greenway Farm, Bath Rd,
Wick, nr. Bath BS30 5RL, UK

ISBN printed book: 978-1-918428-21-6
ISBN e-book: 978-1-918428-22-3

Cover design by Kevin Rylands
Internal design by Mac Style

Printed and bound in the UK

This book is printed on FSC® certified paper

FSC
www.fsc.org
MIX
Paper | Supporting responsible forestry
FSC® C013604

REAL-WORLD CHALLENGES IN CLINICAL MEDICINE

To my daughter, Heather, and her family,
with love and gratitude beyond words.

Contents

Introduction

Clinical medicine is learned best in real practice, where patients rarely present in neat textbook patterns and ideal referral pathways are not always available. Doctors are often required to make important decisions with limited time, incomplete information, and significant system pressures. This book was written to reflect those real-world conditions.

Real-World Challenges in Clinical Medicine presents true clinical cases drawn from everyday practice. Many illustrate situations in which general practitioners in particular, are left managing complex or deteriorating patients in the community because hospital admission is delayed, beds are unavailable, or immediate specialist input cannot be obtained. In these circumstances, clinicians must balance patient safety, clinical judgement, and practical limitations, often in isolation.

Each case demonstrates how careful history-taking, focused examination, structured reasoning, and clear documentation allow safe decision-making even when resources are constrained. The emphasis throughout is on recognising danger signs early, escalating appropriately, and avoiding unnecessary investigations while maintaining patient safety.

The book is intended for **final-year medical students, junior doctors, general practitioners, and frontline clinicians**. Its aim is to strengthen diagnostic confidence, reduce avoidable error and delay, and support safe, cost-effective care. By learning from real cases, readers will develop a pragmatic clinical approach that protects patients while acknowledging the realities of modern healthcare systems, including the NHS.

Note to the Reader. *This book is intended for educational purposes only and does not constitute medical advice or treatment.*

"This book starts where the patient starts —
not where the textbook starts."

Case Study 1

Recurrent Nose Bleeding

This case involved an eleven-year-old boy whom I saw in the mid-1980s. He lived with his parents in their own home. His father worked as a bus driver and his mother was employed as a hospital cleaner. They were a close Afro-Caribbean family, and this boy was their only child. He attended the local school, walked there each day, and was described as a happy and sociable child. There was no history of earlier illness, he was fully immunised, and both parents were non-smokers, providing a stable home environment.

He came to our attention through referral from the ENT department because of recurrent epistaxis. On this occasion the bleeding had been persistent, causing hospital admission and nasal packing. During that admission the ENT surgeon noted that the boy also had abdominal swelling. As this finding was outside his specialty, he referred the patient to the medical team, and I became involved in his care.

Looking back over the history, the nosebleeds had been occurring for several months. The parents had taken him to their general practitioner two or three times. They had been advised on physical measures to control the bleeding, including pinching the nose and applying ice, and told to attend hospital if it did not settle. On several occasions the bleeding had stopped spontaneously, or with these measures.

In the two most recent episodes, however, the epistaxis had been more severe. About a month before the present admission he had required nasal packing in hospital. This time the bleeding once again failed to stop at home and was controlled only after ENT intervention. Because of the additional finding of abdominal enlargement, the case was referred on to medicine.

The boy's past medical history was unremarkable. He had no chronic illnesses, took no regular medication, and had no known allergies. He was growing well and developing normally. There were no family concerns apart from the recurrent nosebleeds.

On examination he looked well and was not pale. There was no petechial rash or purpura. His temperature was 37.1°C and his pulse 100 beats per minute. There was no neck stiffness. Cardiovascular and respiratory examinations were normal, with no murmurs or added sounds.

Abdominal examination, however, revealed clear distension. The liver was palpable about three fingerbreadths below the costal margin, smooth and non-tender. The spleen was not enlarged. There were no bruises, and urine testing at the bedside revealed no blood. His nose was still packed, which limited inspection, but no gross abnormality was noted.

Key Questions

1. **What is the differential diagnosis?**
2. **How should this case be managed?**
3. **What is the final diagnosis?**

The differential diagnosis at this stage was broad. In children, recurrent nosebleeds are usually benign, most often caused by fragile nasal mucosa or minor trauma such as nose-picking. However, the persistence and severity of this boy's bleeding, together with the finding of hepatomegaly, strongly suggested an underlying systemic problem. Platelet dysfunction, such as von Willebrand disease, had to be considered, as did clotting factor deficiencies like haemophilia. Acquired causes of coagulation disturbance, particularly liver disease, became especially important in view of the abdominal findings. Malignancy such as leukaemia was another potential cause, though he looked well and there were no obvious signs of anaemia or bruising.

Management was aimed first at stabilisation and control of the bleeding. He was admitted to hospital and observed closely. The nasal packing was maintained, and supportive measures ensured he remained comfortable. Investigations were then carried out to clarify the underlying cause. These included a full blood count, coagulation profile with bleeding and clotting times, and liver function tests. In addition, screening for viral hepatitis was ordered because of the hepatomegaly.

The results provided the explanation. His haemoglobin and platelet count were normal, which ruled out anaemia and primary platelet deficiency. Bleeding time was also normal, but clotting times were prolonged. Liver function tests were abnormal, and hepatitis B infection was confirmed. This HB unified the picture: the liver enlargement reflected hepatitis B involvement, and the abnormal clotting profile reflected impaired hepatic production of clotting factors. The recurrent epistaxis was therefore a clinical manifestation of disordered coagulation caused by chronic hepatitis B.

With this diagnosis established, the boy was referred to the paediatric gastroenterology team for ongoing care. His immediate bleeding was managed conservatively, while the underlying hepatitis B was investigated and monitored. His parents were counselled, and arrangements were made for screening of close family members, given the possibility of household transmission.

Final Diagnosis

Hepatitis B infection affecting the liver, with impaired clotting function and recurrent bleeding (epistaxis).

Lessons Learned

This case carried several lessons. Nosebleeds in children are common and usually trivial, but recurrent or severe episodes must always prompt consideration of systemic causes. Liver disease, although not often suspected in paediatrics, can present in this subtle way. The ENT surgeon's careful observation of abdominal swelling was pivotal and demonstrates the importance of looking beyond the presenting complaint. Without this observation the diagnosis might have been delayed, with potentially serious consequences.

The case also highlighted the need to consider the family context. Infections such as hepatitis B can affect multiple members of a household, and screening of parents and close relatives is essential. A detailed family history of bleeding disorders or liver disease should also be taken.

For doctors in training, the lesson is to maintain an open mind. Epistaxis is most often benign, but persistence, severity, or association with other abnormalities should trigger a full systemic evaluation. Careful examination, attention to small details such as hepatomegaly, and a willingness to broaden the differential diagnosis are critical. This case illustrates how collaboration across specialties and thorough investigation can lead to the correct diagnosis and appropriate management.

Case Study 2

Fever, Lethargy and Unwell

This case concerned a 52-year-old woman who presented initially to her general practitioner with complaints of weakness, lethargy, low-grade fever, and general malaise. She explained that she had been struggling to carry out her usual daily activities and had noticed a slight but persistent rise in temperature over several days. She had never smoked, drank alcohol only occasionally, and had no significant past medical history. At the time she was not on any regular medication.

At her GP consultation she appeared tired but remained alert and responsive. Her pulse was 100 beats per minute, temperature 37.6°C, blood pressure 135/80 mmHg, and oxygen saturation 98 per cent. Cardiovascular and respiratory examinations were unremarkable, and the GP could not detect any murmurs or added sounds. It must be remembered that in primary care settings, subtle or difficult cardiac murmurs are not always identified, and this limitation is important to recognise. There was no evidence of anaemia, and no neurological deficits were present at this stage.

Routine blood tests were arranged. These showed an erythrocyte sedimentation rate of 51 mm per hour and a C-reactive protein of 40 mg/L, both raised. The full blood count was normal. Liver function was normal, but renal function showed mild disturbance, not sufficient to suggest a specific diagnosis. With no clear abnormalities on examination and only non-specific laboratory findings, the GP concluded that this might represent a viral illness and opted for conservative, supportive management.

Over the following weeks her condition deteriorated. She developed weakness on the right side of her body, affecting both the upper and lower limbs. This was consistent with a cerebrovascular event. She was admitted to her local hospital, where investigations confirmed that she had suffered an embolic stroke.

Echocardiography at that time revealed a murmur consistent with mitral regurgitation, and mitral stenosis was also suspected. She was started on warfarin following confirmation of stroke, treated as a case of bacterial endocarditis though blood cultures were all negative, and initially her neurological symptoms improved.

Unfortunately, this improvement was short-lived. She soon developed recurrent fever, worsening weakness, and urine tests revealed microscopic haematuria. Repeat blood tests showed persistently raised ESR and CRP. Despite being on anticoagulation, she continued to experience further embolic episodes. The ongoing combination of systemic illness, abnormal inflammatory markers, and repeated strokes created a complex diagnostic dilemma.

Key Questions

1. **What do you think is the differential diagnosis?**
2. **How would you manage this case?**
3. **What is the final diagnosis?**

The differential diagnosis at this stage was carefully considered. Infective endocarditis was the leading possibility, as this would account for fever, raised inflammatory markers, microscopic haematuria, and recurrent embolic strokes. Non-bacterial thrombotic endocarditis was another possibility, particularly in the absence of confirmed infection.

Rheumatic mitral valve disease also had to be considered, as it can predispose to embolic events. Systemic vasculitic disorders, with secondary cardiac involvement, were also in the differential. Finally, a primary cardiac tumour such as an atrial myxoma had to be considered, especially given the repeated emboli despite anticoagulation.

She was transferred to a tertiary referral centre in London for further evaluation. By this stage she was on warfarin and taking occasional co-proxamol for pain relief. On admission her investigations again showed persistently high ESR and CRP, microscopic haematuria, normal liver function, and further evidence of embolic strokes.

Advanced echocardiography, including transoesophageal views, revealed a mass attached to the anterior leaflet of the mitral valve. This mass was producing diastolic incompetence and significant regurgitation. The findings raised serious concern, and her case was discussed by a multidisciplinary team including cardiologists, neurologists, and cardiothoracic surgeons. The clinical picture strongly resembled infective endocarditis, but the repeated embolic events despite anticoagulation, combined with the echocardiographic appearance, suggested a tumour.

Given the high risk of ongoing emboli and the uncertainty of diagnosis, surgery was advised. At operation, an atrial myxoma was discovered attached to the anterior leaflet of the mitral valve. The lesion closely resembled endocarditic vegetation, but was excised completely. Histological analysis confirmed it to be a benign cardiac myxoma.

Following surgery, the patient made a remarkable recovery. Her fever settled, inflammatory markers normalised, and with rehabilitation she regained much of her neurological function. She was discharged home in stable condition, with follow-up arranged in both cardiology and neurology clinics.

Final Diagnosis

Left atrial myxoma of the mitral valve, presenting with recurrent embolic strokes and systemic inflammatory features, initially thought to be infective endocarditis.

Lessons Learned

This case illustrates the considerable difficulty in distinguishing between infective endocarditis and cardiac tumours. Fever, high ESR and CRP, haematuria, and embolic strokes all strongly suggested endocarditis. However, the persistence of embolic phenomena despite anticoagulation, together with the absence of microbiological confirmation, should always raise suspicion of alternative causes. The use of advanced echocardiography, especially transoesophageal imaging, was pivotal in detecting the mass. Surgery not only confirmed the diagnosis of atrial myxoma but also provided a cure.

The broader lesson is clear. In any patient presenting with embolic stroke and systemic inflammatory signs, particularly when emboli recur despite treatment, a cardiac tumour must be considered in the differential diagnosis. A narrow focus on infective endocarditis alone could lead to misdiagnosis and delay in definitive treatment. This case underlines the importance of maintaining a broad clinical perspective, of using advanced imaging appropriately, and of timely referral for surgical intervention when indicated.

For medical students and junior doctors, the teaching point is to think beyond the common causes and to remember that not all vegetations on heart valves are infective. Cardiac tumours, although rare, can mimic endocarditis closely, and awareness of this possibility is critical to avoid error. In this case, careful assessment, multidisciplinary discussion, and decisive surgical management together produced an excellent outcome.

Case Study 3

Bilateral Breast Enlargement

This patient was referred to the hospital by his general practitioner, where I first encountered him.

He was a 56-year-old man, married and living with his wife in their own home. He had worked for many years as an accountant, while his wife was employed as a hospital secretary. They had two adult children: a daughter aged 31 who was already in employment, and a son aged 22 who had recently completed his studies and was seeking work. The family described themselves as content and financially secure, and they enjoyed a stable social background without major difficulties.

The patient first attended his general practitioner a few weeks before referral because he had noticed enlargement of both breasts. This change had been gradual in onset, painless, and unaccompanied by nipple discharge. He was, however, embarrassed by the cosmetic alteration and increasingly anxious about its impact on his confidence and intimacy. In addition to these concerns, he admitted that his sexual drive and activity had declined steadily over the preceding months. He denied any history of trauma, orchitis, surgery to the testes, or operations involving the pituitary gland. He had experienced no headaches, visual disturbances, or neurological symptoms which might suggest pituitary pathology.

His past medical history revealed long-standing hypertension that had progressed to congestive cardiac failure, conditions which had required regular follow-up. He had no prior diagnosis of diabetes, thyroid disease, or malignancy.

The drug history proved particularly important. He had been prescribed atenolol, which he had taken for several years for blood pressure control. In addition, he had been taking ranitidine twice daily for the previous four years, following an endoscopically confirmed peptic ulcer. He was also on furosemide 40 mg daily as part of his cardiac management. He had no known drug allergies.

With regard to lifestyle, he admitted to drinking approximately four pints of beer each day. He convinced himself that this intake fell within the safe recommended limits, although in reality it exceeded healthy thresholds and carried significant risks for both hepatic and endocrine function. He denied smoking or taking illicit drugs.

At the initial consultation his general practitioner found him to be well, pleasant, and cooperative. Routine investigations, including renal and liver function tests and a full blood count, were within normal limits. He was reassured and asked to return for review after two months.

On review, however, his breast enlargement had become more obvious. Although still painless and without discharge, it troubled him greatly from a cosmetic point of view, and his sexual function had further deteriorated. Concerned by this progression, the general practitioner referred him for specialist assessment at the hospital.

In the endocrine clinic he was examined in detail. He appeared alert and comfortable. His height was 178 centimetres and his weight 77 kilograms, giving a body mass index within the healthy range. He was not anaemic or cyanosed, and he was not breathless at rest. His pulse was 88 beats per minute, regular in sinus rhythm, and his blood pressure was 145/79 millimetres of mercury. There was no clinical evidence of heart failure: his chest was clear on auscultation, the jugular venous pressure was not raised, and there was no peripheral oedema.

The most striking feature on examination was the gynecomastia. The breast tissue was symmetrically enlarged, smooth in consistency, non-tender, and without discrete lumps or nodules. There was no nipple retraction, no discharge, and no skin dimpling or inflammatory change to suggest malignancy.

The abdomen was soft and non-tender. The liver and spleen were not palpable, and there was no ascites. The testes were of normal size and consistency, without nodularity, atrophy, or tenderness. Neurological examination showed intact visual fields, normal cranial nerves, and no focal deficits. Cardiovascular and respiratory examinations revealed no further abnormality. Overall, the clinical picture pointed more towards an endocrine imbalance rather than a structural lesion such as malignancy.

Key Questions

1. **What are the possible diagnoses and differentials?**
2. **How would you manage this case?**
3. **What was the final diagnosis?**

A number of investigations were arranged. Computed tomography of the head, chest, and abdomen was performed to exclude pathology in the pituitary, testes, or adrenals. A full hormonal profile was requested, including oestrogen, testosterone, and androgens, with additional testing of luteinising hormone, follicle-stimulating hormone, and prolactin. Liver function tests, including gamma-glutamyl transferase, were repeated, together with inflammatory markers such as erythrocyte sedimentation rate and a repeat full blood count.

The results demonstrated low testosterone with raised oestrogen and androgen levels. The computed tomography scans revealed no discrete lesion in the testes, pituitary, or adrenal glands. The liver function tests suggested mild impairment, consistent with early alcohol-related injury, although there was no evidence of cirrhosis.

The differential diagnosis was considered carefully. Drug-induced gynecomastia appeared to be the most likely explanation, since both ranitidine and furosemide are recognised causes of endocrine disturbance.

Alcohol-related hepatic impairment was also a strong contributing factor, as chronic consumption impairs the metabolism of oestrogen and increases circulating levels.

Primary testicular tumours, such as Sertoli or Leydig cell tumours, were considered, but normal examination and imaging made this less likely, though ultrasound was required to exclude them with certainty. Pituitary and adrenal disorders can also produce hormonal imbalance, but in this case the absence of neurological features and normal imaging made these improbable. Idiopathic gynecomastia was a final consideration, though the weight of evidence pointed towards drugs and alcohol.

Management began with a review of medication. Ranitidine was discontinued and replaced with an alternative anti-ulcer therapy. Furosemide, although important in managing his cardiac failure, was reassessed in consultation with his cardiologist to determine if adjustments could be made. Atenolol was less strongly associated with gynecomastia, but remained under review.

Lifestyle modification was a crucial aspect of treatment. The patient was strongly advised to reduce or abstain from alcohol, since his daily consumption of four pints far exceeded healthy limits. He was counselled on the link between alcohol and impaired hormone metabolism, and he accepted the importance of addressing this issue.

Further tests, including testicular ultrasound and more detailed endocrine assays, were recommended to complete the evaluation. If his symptoms of hypogonadism progressed, testosterone replacement therapy could be considered. In severe or persistent gynecomastia, particularly when cosmetic distress was significant, surgical reduction was also discussed as a possible future option.

Regular follow-up with endocrinology and cardiology was arranged, not only to monitor his hormonal and cardiac status but also to provide ongoing support in lifestyle modification.

Lessons Learned

This case highlights the value of a thorough clinical history, especially in relation to prescribed medications and alcohol intake, when evaluating gynecomastia. Many cases can be explained by iatrogenic and lifestyle-related causes, without the need for invasive or costly investigations. Ranitidine, once widely prescribed, is a recognised cause of hormonal disturbance, while loop diuretics such as furosemide have similar potential effects. Chronic alcohol intake further amplifies the problem by impairing hepatic clearance of oestrogens.

Equally important is the psychosocial impact. To the physician, breast enlargement may seem a minor feature, yet for the patient it carried considerable embarrassment and loss of confidence, compounded by declining libido. Addressing the problem required not only clinical reasoning but also sensitivity to the patient's concerns.

For medical students and junior doctors, this case illustrates the importance of beginning with a careful history, considering the common and reversible causes, and using targeted investigations to confirm the diagnosis. Such an approach avoids unnecessary interventions, reduces cost, and most importantly provides timely and effective care.

Case Study 4

Weight Loss, Persistent Diarrhoea for Long Periods

This is the case of a 59-year-old lady who had retired from her teaching job due to ill health. She lived with her husband, a retired car mechanic, in their private home. They had two adult children, aged 32 and 29 years old. The family lived a quiet life and were regular churchgoers, attending services two or three times a week.

She presented to her general practitioner with persistent diarrhoea, which had gradually worsened over time. She also reported progressive weight loss and occasional episodes of blood in the stool. Her appetite remained intact, but she was troubled by bloating and the diarrhoea occurred both day and night, interfering significantly with her daily life.

The GP arranged preliminary investigations and referred her to hospital. Initial tests showed evidence of malabsorption, with deficiencies in fat-soluble vitamins, hypocalcaemia, and iron deficiency anaemia. She was started on oral iron therapy. An upper gastrointestinal endoscopy was performed, but no gross lesion was identified. Small-bowel biopsies were taken, although the outcome was inconclusive. This took place in 1978, when diagnostic resources were more limited than today. She was discharged with calcium and iron supplements, together with a referral to the dietician.

Her past medical history was significant. She had never smoked and drank alcohol only occasionally, perhaps one or two pints of beer in an entire week. She suffered from long-standing rheumatoid arthritis, which had been difficult to control and had led to her early retirement. The disease caused multi-organ involvement and severe joint deformities, particularly in her hands, elbows, and knees.

Over the years she had received repeated courses of systemic steroids as well as intra-articular injections. At the age of 44 she had also undergone hysterectomy for excessive uterine bleeding. At the time of this illness, her regular medications included naproxen and ranitidine, which provided only partial relief.

Her condition deteriorated, and she was referred again to hospital. By this stage she had lost considerable weight and was increasingly weak. She had also developed exertional breathlessness.

On admission I saw her personally. She looked pale but was not jaundiced or cyanosed. At rest she was not breathless. Her weight was 62 kilograms, noticeably underweight for her tall frame of 170 centimetres. Her temperature was 37.1°C, her pulse 100 beats per minute in sinus rhythm, and her blood pressure 110 over 70 millimetres of mercury.

Cardiovascular examination revealed normal heart sounds with no murmurs or rubs. The chest was clear to auscultation, with no added sounds, no effusion, and no chest wall nodules. The abdomen was soft and non-tender. The liver was palpable three centimetres below the costal margin, smooth and non-tender. The spleen was also enlarged, two fingerbreadths below the costal margin, smooth and non-tender, with no evidence of ascites.

Examination of the joints confirmed long-standing rheumatoid arthritis, with marked ulnar deviation of both hands and deformities of the elbows and knees. No acute effusion was present. Neurological examination showed no peripheral neuropathy, cranial nerves were intact, and there were no abnormal neurological findings.

Key Questions

1. **What are the possible diagnoses and differentials?**
2. **How would you manage this case?**
3. **What was the final diagnosis?**

The clinical picture pointed to a wide range of possibilities. Chronic diarrhoea, weight loss, bloating, and anaemia naturally raised concerns about malignancy of the colon. Inflammatory bowel disease, such as Crohn's disease or ulcerative colitis, was also possible. Coeliac disease and pancreatic insufficiency could not be excluded. Infective diarrhoea seemed less likely, given the prolonged course. The combination of hepatosplenomegaly, anaemia, malabsorption, and her background of rheumatoid arthritis, however, strongly suggested a systemic disorder.

Investigations were pursued systematically. Blood tests, including renal and liver function, inflammatory markers, calcium, vitamin levels, and iron profile, were repeated to assess the extent of malabsorption. Stool studies excluded infection. Abdominal imaging confirmed hepatosplenomegaly, but showed no mass lesions. Colonoscopy with biopsy ruled out malignancy and inflammatory bowel disease. Repeat small-bowel biopsies were performed, and histology revealed amyloid deposition in the intestinal mucosa. Urinalysis supported this diagnosis, demonstrating heavy proteinuria consistent with renal amyloid involvement.

The evidence confirmed secondary amyloidosis, secondary to poorly-controlled rheumatoid arthritis, with multi-organ involvement affecting the gastrointestinal tract, liver, spleen, and kidneys.

Final Diagnosis

Secondary amyloidosis, secondary to rheumatoid arthritis, with systemic involvement of the gastrointestinal tract, liver, spleen, and kidneys.

Lessons Learned

This case demonstrated how chronic inflammatory disease can lead to devastating systemic complications. Rheumatoid arthritis is often considered primarily in terms of joint destruction, yet in reality it also carries the risk of multi-organ damage when inadequately controlled. Continuous inflammation leads to overproduction of serum amyloid A protein, which deposits in tissues and results in secondary amyloidosis.

The presentation of diarrhoea, weight loss, and anaemia could easily have been attributed to more common gastrointestinal conditions such as malignancy, inflammatory bowel disease, or coeliac disease. The presence of hepatosplenomegaly and proteinuria, however, provided crucial clues to the systemic nature of her illness. This case emphasises the importance of considering the whole clinical picture, integrating findings across multiple systems, rather than focusing only on isolated symptoms.

From a management perspective, the key lies in aggressive treatment of the underlying inflammatory disease. In modern practice, disease-modifying anti-rheumatic drugs and biologic therapies have greatly reduced the incidence of secondary amyloidosis. In the 1970s, however, treatment options were limited, and reliance on corticosteroids and non-steroidal drugs was often inadequate. Supportive measures such as nutritional supplementation and management of renal involvement remain important, although once amyloidosis is established, complete reversal is rarely possible.

For final-year medical students and junior doctors, this case provides an important lesson in diagnostic reasoning. It illustrates the need to think beyond common gastrointestinal disorders when faced with chronic diarrhoea and malabsorption, particularly in a patient with long-standing inflammatory disease. It also highlights the value of detailed history-taking, thorough examination, and the integration of systemic findings in order to arrive at the correct diagnosis.

Case Study 5

Palpitations

This is the case of a 49-year-old gentleman who was referred by his general practitioner with a history of palpitations.

He had worked for many years as a bus driver, a steady occupation with long hours and responsibility. He was married, and his wife was employed as a shop assistant. Together they had two grown-up children, aged 22 and 20, both in higher education. The family lived in a terraced house in suburban London and enjoyed a settled, happy life.

According to his history, the palpitations had been present for about three months before he consulted his GP. He described them as a sensation of his heart thumping in his chest. They tended to occur during exertion, such as climbing stairs or washing the car, but settled with rest. At first, he paid little attention to them, but over time he became increasingly concerned and anxious. On some occasions he noticed very mild chest discomfort, though this was vague and non-specific.

At his first consultation, the GP examined him thoroughly. According to the referral letter, his blood pressure was measured, thyroid examined, and a full neurological and mental assessment performed. No abnormality was found. The GP reassured him, advised him to relax and spend more time socially with his family, and suggested he return if symptoms persisted.

A few weeks later the palpitations recurred and he returned to the surgery. Once again no abnormality was detected. In the meantime, baseline investigations had been carried out, including thyroid function tests, full blood count, renal function, and liver function. All were normal. The GP also noted that the palpitations never occurred during sleep. An

ECG was requested from the hospital, which showed normal sinus rhythm with no evidence of ischaemia or arrhythmia.

His social history revealed that he never smoked and drank only a couple of pints of beer each week. He had no significant past medical history, apart from an appendicectomy in his youth. He was not taking any regular medication and had no known allergies.

On referral to hospital, I assessed him personally. He was a well-built man, standing 177 centimetres tall and weighing 75 kilograms. Examination of the thyroid revealed no enlargement and no features of thyrotoxicosis. His eyes were normal, with no exophthalmos. His pulse was 94 beats per minute in sinus rhythm, and his blood pressure was 140/90 mmHg. Heart sounds were normal, with no murmurs or added sounds. His chest was clear, with vesicular breath sounds and no added sounds. The trachea was central. His abdomen was soft and non-tender, with no organomegaly. Neurological examination, including cranial nerves and both upper and lower limbs, was normal. There was no tremor. Mentally he was alert, cooperative, and pleasant, though understandably anxious about his symptoms.

I explained to him that further investigations were needed. Repeat thyroid function tests, including thyroid antibodies, were requested to exclude early thyrotoxicosis. Full blood count was repeated to rule out anaemia, and renal and liver functions were reassessed. All results came back normal.

Key Questions

1. **What is the differential diagnosis?**
2. **What is the appropriate action plan for further investigation and management?**
3. **What was the final diagnosis?**

The differential diagnosis was broad. Palpitations are a common symptom and may be caused by arrhythmias, endocrine disorders, anaemia, structural heart disease, or psychological stress. Thyrotoxicosis was an important consideration, but repeated thyroid tests were normal. Anaemia was excluded by normal haemoglobin and indices. Structural heart disease seemed less likely in the absence of murmurs or abnormal ECG findings. Hypertension was present but not severe. Psychological stress or anxiety remained a strong possibility, particularly given the absence of abnormalities on investigation and the clear link between exertion and awareness of his heartbeat. Functional palpitations, related to heightened autonomic awareness, were also considered.

The next step was prolonged rhythm monitoring. A Holter monitor was arranged to record his heart activity over a 24-hour period. This was particularly useful because he reported that palpitations occurred mainly during exertion. The Holter recording showed a normal rhythm throughout, with no arrhythmias or episodes of tachycardia. His pulse simply increased appropriately during physical activity and returned to normal at rest and during sleep. There was no evidence of supraventricular tachycardia, atrial fibrillation, or ventricular ectopy.

This finding was highly reassuring. It demonstrated that his palpitations were not due to structural heart disease or pathological arrhythmias, but rather represented a normal physiological response magnified by heightened awareness and anxiety.

When reviewed in clinic after the Holter results, I discussed the findings in detail with him. I explained that his heart was structurally normal, with no abnormal rhythms, and that the palpitations were most likely stress-related. I emphasised that this was a common problem in modern life, often aggravated by occupational pressures.

He accepted this explanation, but admitted that the palpitations continued to trouble him. He asked whether anything could help him feel calmer. After discussion, a short course of diazepam 2 mg was prescribed, to be taken once to three times daily as required. I cautioned him not to exceed the dose, especially because of his work as a bus driver, and emphasised that he should not drive if he felt sedated.

He was discharged back to his GP with advice on lifestyle modification, including relaxation, stress reduction, and sleep hygiene.

Final Diagnosis

Functional palpitations related to stress and anxiety, without evidence of cardiac pathology.

Lessons Learned

This case illustrates the complexity of assessing palpitations. While arrhythmias and heart disease must always be excluded, many cases are benign. Functional palpitations, often associated with anxiety and heightened awareness of the normal heartbeat, are common but can cause significant distress.

It also highlights the importance of systematic investigation. Thyroid disease, anaemia, and biochemical abnormalities were excluded. Electrocardiography showed no abnormality. Holter monitoring provided definitive reassurance by confirming normal rhythm throughout. This structured approach allowed us to reach a safe and confident conclusion.

Equally important was communication and empathy. The patient's symptoms were genuine and worrying for him, even in the absence of pathology. Explaining the findings carefully, involving him in the reasoning, and offering supportive treatment helped to alleviate his anxiety.

For medical students and junior doctors, this case reinforces the principle that palpitations are not always cardiac in origin. A thorough history, appropriate investigation, and sensitivity to psychological factors are essential. Above all, reassurance must be based on evidence, not assumption. Careful explanation and a supportive approach are as important as the investigations themselves.

Case Study 6

Right Abdomen Pain and Vomiting

This patient, a 71-year-old man, had generally enjoyed reasonable health for his age. He lived with his wife and son, while his three grown daughters lived independently. He led a simple, pleasant lifestyle, often spending time in cafés or sitting by the beach. He had never smoked and did not drink alcohol.

Within the space of a single day he became acutely unwell. He developed a high temperature and began to vomit, though there was no diarrhoea. He also experienced pain in the right upper abdomen. Hoping it would settle, he took paracetamol, but there was no improvement. He then noticed the sudden appearance of deep jaundice and dark urine. Recognising the seriousness of these signs, he presented to hospital and was admitted urgently.

His past health included gallstones, which had caused occasional flare-ups over the years. These had been managed conservatively with analgesics and occasional antibiotics, without the need for surgery. He also had type 2 diabetes controlled with diet and metformin, and hypertension for which he took losartan. In addition, he had benign prostatic hyperplasia, which caused few symptoms and required no treatment. He reported no drug allergies.

On admission he looked acutely unwell and confused. His temperature was 38.9°C, pulse 120 beats per minute, blood pressure 140/90 mmHg, and his breathing was rapid. Oxygen saturation was slightly reduced. His chest was clear with vesicular breath sounds, and cardiovascular examination revealed no murmurs. His abdomen was tender in the right upper quadrant. His weight was 90 kilograms and height 179 centimetres.

Key Questions

1. **What is your differential diagnosis?**
2. **How do you manage it?**
3. **What is the final diagnosis?**

In an elderly man with fever, confusion, right upper abdominal pain, jaundice, and a known history of gallstones, the differential diagnosis centres on the hepatobiliary system. Acute cholecystitis with systemic sepsis is a strong possibility, especially given his gallstone history. Acute cholangitis is another leading consideration, particularly as the triad of fever, jaundice, and abdominal pain – Charcot's triad – was evident, with confusion suggesting Reynolds' pentad and severe infection. Common bile duct obstruction by a gallstone must also be considered, as this may precipitate ascending cholangitis. A liver abscess could present with fever and pain, but would usually be more insidious. Severe viral hepatitis remains a differential, though the rapid onset with sepsis makes it less likely here.

The management of such a case requires immediate admission and aggressive treatment. Intravenous broad-spectrum antibiotics are essential, initiated promptly and later tailored once culture results are available. In this patient, blood cultures grew Escherichia coli, guiding therapy. Intravenous fluids are needed to support circulation and prevent renal compromise. A central venous line allows careful monitoring of fluid balance and administration of therapy.

A bladder catheter is placed to measure urine output, providing an important marker of renal perfusion and septic severity. Urea and electrolytes must be checked frequently. Imaging is crucial to determine whether there is ongoing obstruction or residual collection. Ultrasound may show gallstones or bile duct dilatation, while CT or MRI can provide further definition. Endoscopic retrograde cholangiopancreatography

(ERCP) may be required if there is obstruction of the common bile duct, both to diagnose and to relieve blockage.

Lesson Learned

This case demonstrates the potentially life-threatening nature of cholangitis. The classic triad of jaundice, fever, and abdominal pain was present, and his confusion added evidence of severe sepsis. Even after cholecystectomy, infection persisted within the biliary system, reminding us that surgery does not always eradicate the source if bacteria have entered the ducts.

The relapse following early discharge emphasises the importance of prolonged intravenous antibiotic therapy and inpatient observation until recovery is secure. Premature transition to oral antibiotics risks recurrence, as was seen here. Repeat imaging is vital whenever progress is incomplete, to identify residual infection or obstruction.

The lesson is clear: cholangitis demands vigilance, careful multi-disciplinary management, and close follow-up. Only with sustained therapy and monitoring can relapse and serious complications be avoided.

Final Diagnosis

Acute cholangitis.

In this patient, the hospital team first diagnosed acute gallbladder infection and proceeded with cholecystectomy. Post-operatively, however, his fever persisted, his jaundice deepened, and he remained confused. He was treated with intravenous antibiotics, adjusted once blood cultures identified E coli. Supportive care was continued with intravenous fluids, central monitoring, bladder catheterisation, and careful biochemical follow-up. For the first three days his temperature remained high, but on the fourth day his condition began to improve. His temperature settled, urine output increased, and his confusion cleared. He was discharged after a week, prescribed oral antibiotics, and felt better at the time of discharge.

Three days later, however, he relapsed. His temperature rose again and he felt generally unwell, although his jaundice was improving. Repeat imaging with CT and MRI revealed residual infection within the biliary system. He was re-admitted, given further intravenous antibiotics for five days, and closely observed. Gradually he improved, with resolution of fever and stabilisation of his condition, allowing safe discharge once more.

Case Study 7

Progressive Shortness of Breath

This case concerns a 58-year-old gentleman, originally from Saudi Arabia who divided his time between that country and Britain. He had lived for many years in Saudi Arabia, where his business interests were based, but regularly spent several months in Britain each year to manage his affairs and oversee his children's education. His family resided mostly in Britain, as his children were enrolled in schools and universities there.

He was married with four children, all of them grown or nearly grown. He had never consumed alcohol, but he had smoked between ten and fifteen cigarettes daily for more than thirty years. He denied any recreational drug use.

He was referred to hospital by his general practitioner with a history of vague but troubling symptoms. He complained of mild breathlessness on exertion, together with persistent fatigue and a general sense of sluggishness. He tired easily and was no longer able to travel independently, something he had once done routinely. He denied chest pain, palpitations, significant weight loss, vomiting, or gastrointestinal symptoms.

His GP had found no specific abnormality but, recognising that the complaints were non-specific yet concerning, referred him for specialist assessment. At the time, I was working as a medical registrar in general medicine, and I became involved in his care.

His past medical history included removal of the right testicle many years earlier in Saudi Arabia. According to his account, the testis had become gangrenous following severe orchitis, though no documentation was available. Two years before this admission, he had been treated for a urinary tract infection in Saudi Arabia. At that time, investigations including calcium levels and prostate-specific antigen were said to be normal. He was not taking any regular medication and had no known allergies.

On assessment, he appeared intelligent, articulate, and comfortable at rest. He had no cough or wheeze, and was not cyanosed or clinically anaemic. His height was 178 centimetres and his weight 80 kilograms. His pulse was irregular at 94 beats per minute, consistent with atrial fibrillation. The jugular venous pressure was raised to eight centimetres, with obvious pulsation visible in the neck.

Palpation of the praecordium made localisation of the apex beat difficult. Heart sounds were soft but without a distinct murmur or pericardial rub. Respiratory examination revealed a central trachea and no clubbing. Chest expansion was generally reduced, with vesicular breath sounds overall but diminished at the left base, suggesting an effusion.

Examination of the abdomen showed mild distension. The liver edge was palpable three centimetres below the costal margin, smooth and non-tender. The spleen was not palpable. There was a small degree of ascites suggested on clinical grounds. Both ankles were swollen with bilateral oedema. Neurological examination was normal. He was alert, cooperative, and fully oriented.

Key Questions

1. **What is the differential diagnosis in this case?**
2. **What is the appropriate plan of action to proceed with investigation and management?**
3. **What was the final diagnosis?**

The presenting features were non-specific but clearly concerning. The combination of lethargy, mild breathlessness on exertion, raised jugular venous pressure, peripheral oedema, hepatomegaly, ascites, muffled heart sounds, and basal effusion suggested cardiac involvement, most likely right-sided heart failure. The irregular pulse confirmed atrial fibrillation, which could be either a primary rhythm disorder or secondary to underlying structural disease.

The differential diagnosis included pericardial effusion with or without tamponade, constrictive pericarditis, cardiomyopathy, ischaemic heart disease, and pulmonary hypertension. Tuberculosis was an important consideration, given his background and travel history. Malignancy, whether primary or metastatic, was another possible cause. Autoimmune and collagen vascular disorders also needed to be kept in mind, particularly if pericardial involvement was secondary.

Initial investigations were arranged. A chest X-ray was requested to assess cardiac size and possible pleural effusion. An ECG confirmed atrial fibrillation and suggested low voltage complexes, which raised the suspicion of pericardial effusion. Blood tests included a full blood count, ESR, renal and liver function, and autoantibody screening. Results showed normal haemoglobin and white cell count. The ESR was raised at 35 mm/hour, and the CRP was 30 mg/L. Renal function was preserved apart from mild proteinuria (2+). Liver function was within normal limits.

At this stage the patient was stable and not in immediate danger. He requested to return home for a week before further admission, which was agreed. When he came back, the district hospital where I was working lacked the resources for advanced cardiac investigation and management of suspected pericardial disease. He was therefore referred to the nearby university hospital, which had the facilities and expertise required.

At the university hospital, further investigations confirmed a large pericardial effusion. Pericardiocentesis was performed, and the aspirated fluid was sent for cytology and microbiology. Both were negative, with no evidence of malignancy or bacterial infection. Given his background, risk factors, and positive Mantoux test, tuberculosis was considered the most likely diagnosis.

He was treated with diuretics to relieve fluid overload, digoxin for rate control of atrial fibrillation, and commenced on empirical antituberculous therapy. Screening of his family members was arranged as a precaution. Over the following months his condition improved remarkably. His breathlessness resolved, his energy levels returned, and he regained normal functional capacity. Continued outpatient follow-up confirmed sustained improvement.

Final Diagnosis

Probable tuberculous pericardial effusion with secondary right-sided heart failure and atrial fibrillation.

Lessons Learned

This case illustrates several important teaching points. First, vague complaints such as lethargy and mild breathlessness on exertion can conceal serious underlying disease. Careful clinical examination, including assessment of jugular venous pressure, heart sounds, hepatomegaly, and peripheral oedema, revealed strong evidence of cardiac involvement before advanced investigations were undertaken.

Second, pericardial effusion is a condition that frequently requires referral to a specialist centre. A district hospital may detect the signs and initiate management, but pericardiocentesis and definitive diagnosis often demand tertiary-level expertise. Recognising the limits of one's resources and referring promptly is crucial.

Third, negative cytology and microbiology do not rule out tuberculosis. Clinical judgment, epidemiological context, and therapeutic response often play a decisive role. In this patient, the absence of malignancy, a positive Mantoux test, and his clinical improvement on antituberculous therapy together confirmed the working diagnosis.

Finally, tuberculosis remains an important cause of pericardial disease in patients from endemic regions. Screening of close family contacts is essential.

For students and junior doctors, the key lesson is to integrate history, examination, and investigation carefully, remain alert to subtle systemic clues, and know when to escalate care to a higher-level centre.

Case Study 8

Childhood Murmur and COPD

This is a 48-year-old Romanian lady who attended our practice for a new-patient examination. She had been living in the United Kingdom for approximately three years at the time of registration. She is single and has one son, aged 22, who remains in Romania. Since her arrival she has been employed as a packer in a local factory, a role she continues to maintain.

Her English is limited, and communication during the consultation required patience, repetition, and the use of simple words. Despite this, she was cooperative and able to convey her background and medical history. She resides in shared accommodation with other tenants and had recently moved into our practice catchment area from another part of the country.

Her past medical history was notable for an earlier ectopic pregnancy, which had required hospital admission and intervention some years earlier. She reported no other significant illnesses but did confirm that she has smoked regularly for the past 20 years. This history of chronic tobacco use is relevant to her present condition.

The new-patient consultation began as routine. She did not present with active complaints, denying chest pain, palpitations, fainting episodes, or leg swelling. She stated that she was able to continue her factory work without significant restriction.

On general examination she appeared of average build and in no acute distress. Her pulse rate was 95 beats per minute, regular, and her blood pressure was within the normal range (125/75 mmHg). Respiratory rate and temperature were also normal. There were no signs of anaemia or jaundice. Peripheral pulses were palpable, and no ankle oedema was present.

When the lungs were auscultated, there were findings consistent with chronic obstructive pulmonary disease (COPD). This has been confirmed by spirometry, with an FEV1/FVC ratio of 62 per cent. She had diffuse wheeze and diminished breath sounds in parts of both lung fields. These changes correlated with her long smoking history. Importantly, she also demonstrated early cyanosis, particularly in the lips and fingers, raising concern about long-standing hypoxia.

On auscultation of the heart a systolic murmur was detected. At this point she volunteered that she had, in fact, been told about the presence of a murmur since childhood. It had apparently been mentioned to her by doctors in Romania, but she had never undergone further assessment and no treatment had been offered. The murmur was soft, without obvious radiation or thrill, but in the context of her overall clinical picture it could not be considered trivial. Both the first and second heart sounds were otherwise present, though somewhat obscured by her chest findings.

The discovery of the murmur, already known since childhood, together with the appearance of cyanosis and the background of COPD, raises important clinical considerations. This is not simply the incidental finding of an innocent murmur. The coexistence of a congenital or long-standing structural lesion with the added burden of chronic lung disease means her case requires careful investigation and follow-up.

Key Questions

1. **What do you think the differential diagnosis of this case is?**
2. **What is your action plan for this patient?**
3. **What is the final diagnosis?**

Baseline investigations were therefore arranged. Blood tests included a full blood count, renal and liver function, thyroid profile, and glucose. These were not only to exclude common reversible factors but also to establish baseline health in a patient with both cardiac and respiratory concerns. A chest radiograph was requested to assess lung hyperinflation, cardiac size, and pulmonary vasculature. An ECG was ordered to check for right-sided strain, conduction abnormalities, or atrial enlargement. Most importantly, an echocardiogram referral was made to evaluate her cardiac valves, chamber sizes, and to clarify the source of the murmur.

As the attending GP, I aimed to complete as much of the basic assessment as possible before onward referral, so that secondary care would already have the essential information at hand. These investigations were organised promptly, and the patient has now been referred to cardiology for specialist assessment.

Interpreter support was organised for her investigations and future appointments, given her limited English. It was explained in simple terms that she had a heart murmur that doctors had known about since her childhood, and that now, combined with her smoking-related chest disease and the signs of low oxygen, it needed to be looked at carefully. Written notes were provided, and the importance of attending her appointments was emphasised.

She was also given advice about potential symptoms which might require earlier medical review, including worsening breathlessness, chest pain, fainting, ankle swelling, or any episodes of fever with worsening cough. Her smoking history was addressed directly, and advice on cessation was provided. She was made aware of local support services for quitting smoking, and this was strongly encouraged as a measure that could benefit both her lung disease and overall cardiovascular health.

It was also explained that not all murmurs are dangerous. Some remain stable and require no specific treatment beyond monitoring. However, the combination of her past and present findings made further assessment essential. She accepted this explanation and agreed to attend the echocardiogram.

The outcome of investigations would determine future management. If the echocardiogram confirmed a benign murmur with no structural abnormality, reassurance and periodic monitoring would suffice. However, if a congenital lesion, valvular disease, or evidence of right-sided cardiac strain was demonstrated, it would be managed in the hospital. The management of her COPD would also need to be optimised, as the interplay between chronic lung disease and cardiac health is significant.

Final Diagnosis

A right-to-left reversal of a previous congenital heart disease - atrial septal defect - aggravated by COPD with central cyanosis.

Lessons Learned

This case highlights the importance of listening carefully to the patient's history, even when language barriers exist. The fact that she had been told about a murmur since childhood altered the interpretation entirely. What might have seemed like an incidental new finding was in fact part of a long-standing condition, possibly congenital, which had never been fully investigated. The presence of cyanosis and COPD further complicates the picture, demonstrating the interplay between chronic lung disease and the cardiovascular system.

The case also underscores the need for careful communication with patients whose first language is not English. Interpreter support, patience, and clear explanations are essential. Finally, it illustrates the role of the GP in not only detecting clinical signs but also piecing together a lifetime of history to form a coherent plan of investigation and management.

Case Study 9

Forgetfulness

This patient was an 82-year-old married man who had been registered at the practice for more than thirty years. A retired soldier, he lived alone in a bungalow following the death of his wife. He attended the surgery regularly, often to collect prescriptions, but also to maintain some social contact and break the isolation of living alone. Over the preceding two years he had begun to show signs of forgetfulness, which he himself occasionally acknowledged. He told me more than once that he noticed he was 'getting a bit muddled,' but he insisted he was coping and relied on writing reminder notes for himself. The practice kept a close watch, and it became increasingly clear that his mental powers were gradually declining month by month.

His social history was notable for a daily alcohol intake of two pints of beer. He smoked one pack of cigarettes a day and had done so for more than thirty years, a habit that began in the army when cigarettes were freely provided. His medications at the time included atenolol 50 mg once daily, Adalat 10 mg three times a day (a calcium-channel blocker), and a salbutamol inhaler, two puffs as required. He reported an allergy to nitrofurantoin, prescribed many years earlier for a urinary tract infection related to a kidney stone.

On physical examination he was 173 centimetres tall and weighed 78 kilograms. His blood pressure on medication was stable at 140/63 mmHg. Heart sounds were normal, with no added sounds. The trachea was central, there was no clubbing, and occasional wheeze was heard scattered across the chest. His temperature was normal. Neurologically he was grossly intact, with normal tone, power, reflexes, sensation and coordination in both upper and lower limbs. Abdominal examination showed no active problems, no tenderness, and no palpable organ enlargement.

At his daughter's request I brought him in for a more detailed assessment. A mini-mental state examination placed him on the borderline of the acceptable range. To exclude reversible causes, I arranged routine investigations: syphilis serology, vitamin B12, folate, renal function, liver function, and a full blood count including mean corpuscular volume. All results came back within normal limits.

Despite these reassuring blood results, his memory continued to deteriorate. Twice he left taps running overnight until his daughter discovered them the following morning. His short-term memory was clearly impaired, although in conversation his judgement and insight still seemed relatively preserved.

At one consultation I advised him that it was no longer safe for him to drive. He resisted strongly, insisting that the car was essential to his life – vital for shopping, visiting friends, going to the pub, and attending church. I listened and acknowledged his feelings but explained that public safety had to come first. He abruptly cut short the discussion with a dismissive, 'I'll take on what you're saying, doc,' but the impression was clear that he had no intention of giving up driving.

A month later the police contacted the practice. He had been found lost at the wheel, confused and disoriented, unable to remember how to get back home. I discussed the case with the police and informed his daughter. She shared her concern, but admitted he was stubborn and unyielding. We called him back for a further discussion, warning him that continued driving would inevitably lead to police involvement. He dismissed this bluntly, declaring that no one could take his car away.

The matter escalated further. He returned to the surgery the following day and threatened staff and doctors with physical assault if anyone attempted to remove his driving privileges. This behaviour caused real fear among staff, who suddenly found themselves in a difficult position

– caring for an elderly patient with dementia, but also facing threats and intimidation. The police were informed, as they were already aware of his difficulties.

I spoke to him again, appealing directly to his sense of reason, practically begging him to stop driving. He appeared to relent, promising that he would give up driving. Yet only a month later, the police again found him lost in his car, disoriented and confused, still continuing to drive despite repeated warnings from myself, his daughter, and the authorities.

At this point the question becomes unavoidable: what would you do in this situation?

This case illustrates a very real dilemma for general practitioners and hospital doctors alike. An elderly patient with progressive cognitive impairment poses a risk to himself and to the public by continuing to drive. He has ignored advice from his family, disregarded medical warnings, been found lost and disoriented by the police on more than one occasion, and has even escalated to threatening violence against healthcare staff. His autonomy and desire to remain independent are in direct conflict with the duty of the doctor to protect wider society.

The professional and legal framework provides guidance. The General Medical Council (GMC) is clear that while patient confidentiality is fundamental, it is not absolute. When a patient's behaviour places others at serious risk of harm, doctors may disclose relevant information without consent. The GMC explicitly addresses the issue of driving: patients with conditions that impair safe driving must inform the Driver and Vehicle Licensing Agency (DVLA). Doctors should advise them of this duty. If the patient refuses to notify the DVLA, and continues to drive, the doctor has a responsibility to breach confidentiality and inform the DVLA directly, explaining to the patient why this step has been taken. In other words, protecting the public overrides the obligation of confidentiality.

The DVLA itself requires patients to stop driving and inform them of any medical condition likely to impair driving ability. Failure to do so is a breach of the law. Where dementia or cognitive decline is involved, doctors play a critical role in identifying risk. If persuasion fails, the responsibility shifts: it is no longer optional for the doctor but mandatory, under professional duty, to notify the DVLA in the interests of public safety.

This case also raised an additional safeguarding concern: the safety of healthcare staff. Threats of physical violence cannot be ignored, even when they come from an elderly or cognitively impaired patient. Every incident must be carefully documented, reported to senior colleagues, and shared with the police if there is credible risk. Protecting staff, other patients, and the practice premises is part of the wider safeguarding duty. The NHS cannot provide care if its workforce is intimidated or unsafe.

What makes this case particularly memorable is how quickly a medical issue - forgetfulness and early dementia - evolved into a multi-layered problem involving the law, regulatory bodies, safeguarding, and public protection. It demonstrated vividly that medicine does not exist in isolation. Doctors are not only diagnosticians but also advocates, protectors, and, when necessary, enforcers of public safety.

Driving is not simply a practical matter for elderly patients; it symbolises independence, freedom, and dignity. Removing that right can feel deeply cruel. Yet, as this case shows, the consequences of allowing an unfit driver to continue are potentially catastrophic. The balance between compassion for the individual and duty to society is delicate, but when life and safety are at risk, the decision must always be clear.

For me, the lessons from this case were stark. First, that documentation at every stage is essential - both the clinical assessments and the behavioural incidents must be recorded in detail. Second, that communication with the patient and the family, however strained, must continue, offering every opportunity for voluntary compliance. Third, that when persuasion fails, the doctor must act decisively - inform the DVLA, work with the police, and take steps to protect staff. And finally, that dementia, while often thought of as a private decline, can spill into public spaces with consequences which affect the whole community.

This was not an easy case to manage, and it left a lasting impression on me. It reminded me that the role of the doctor is not confined to the consultation room. It extends to protecting society, safeguarding colleagues, and sometimes making the hard decisions that patients resist.

Final Diagnosis

Cognitive decline with progressive memory impairment (early dementia), unfit to drive, persistent non-compliance with advice, associated with threats towards healthcare staff and continued risk to public safety.

Case Study 10

Mid-Back Pain

A 55-year-old man, originally from the Middle East, had emigrated to the United Kingdom 20 years earlier and was employed as a hospital porter. He was married with two children aged 16 and 18. He had never smoked, did not drink alcohol, and had been in reasonably good health until the onset of his current problem.

Approximately 12 months before presentation, he developed mid-back pain. Initially, he managed his symptoms at home with paracetamol, which gave him some relief, but over time the pain became more persistent and the analgesia lost its effect. He did not experience any bowel or bladder disturbance, no alteration in sensation, and no systemic symptoms such as weight loss or night sweats. After several months he sought medical advice from his general practitioner.

On his first visit, the GP found no abnormality on examination and prescribed co-proxamol. The patient noted slight improvement but the pain soon returned. At a subsequent review, the GP again found no significant clinical signs. He advised continuation of co-proxamol and added a non-steroidal anti-inflammatory drug. A plain radiograph of the thoracic and lumbar spine was arranged and reported as showing no obvious abnormality. The patient was reassured and advised to persist with analgesia, but as his symptoms did not improve, he was eventually referred to hospital, where I assessed him.

His past medical history was notable for pulmonary tuberculosis diagnosed eight years earlier, successfully treated in hospital with no evidence of recurrence. He also suffered from hypertension, controlled with atenolol 50 mg once daily, and had benign prostatic hypertrophy, managed conservatively without medication.

Basic investigations at this stage included a full blood count, which was normal, an erythrocyte sedimentation rate of 30 mm/hr, and normal renal and liver function. The plain radiograph of the spine once again showed no abnormality.

Key Questions

1. **What is the differential diagnosis, and which is the most likely one?**
2. **How would you manage this case?**

At this point, the important question was the underlying cause of his persistent pain. In a patient of this profile, the differential diagnosis is broad. Infection must always be considered. A pyogenic spinal abscess can present in this way, but in this particular patient, tuberculosis of the spine (Pott's disease) was a strong possibility given his previous history.

Neoplastic disease is another important category. Primary spinal tumours are rare, but metastatic deposits in the spine are relatively common, particularly from primary malignancies of the lung, breast, prostate, or kidney. A rarer entity, yet not to be forgotten, is an ependymoma of the spinal cord, which can also present with progressive back pain. In this case, ependymoma was considered the most likely diagnosis, although infection and metastatic disease could not be excluded at the outset.

Management of such a case must begin with the recognition that persistent mid-back pain lasting for weeks or months is never trivial and must be investigated. A plain radiograph, though useful, is often entirely normal in the early stages of serious disease. But in 1981, the MRI scan was not available, and the best approach at that time was to rely on a CT scan and myelogram in order to identify the underlying problem. Blood investigations, including inflammatory markers, were helpful but could not be relied upon alone.

Referral to a specialist service was essential, whether to orthopaedics, neurology, or neurosurgery, depending on the evolving findings. Most crucially, the appearance of any compression symptoms, such as weakness, sensory disturbance, or bowel and bladder dysfunction, had to be treated as an emergency, as these often indicated spinal cord compression requiring urgent neurosurgical attention.

Final Diagnosis

Ependymoma of the spinal cord presenting with persistent mid-back pain.

Comment

This case illustrates not only the importance of clinical vigilance but also the evolution of medical technology over time. In the early 1980s, the absence of MRI limited the ability to visualise the spine directly, and clinicians had to rely on CT scanning and invasive myelography to reach a diagnosis. Today, MRI is widely available and has become the gold standard for assessing spinal pathology, offering unparalleled detail and eliminating the risks associated with older techniques. Comparing past practice with current standards highlights the progress made in diagnostic imaging and underlines the continuing need for careful clinical judgement when evaluating back pain.

Lesson Learned

The learning points from this case are clear. Persistent mid-back pain lasting more than a few weeks must be taken seriously and investigated thoroughly. The important possibilities include spinal infection, whether pyogenic or tuberculous, as well as both primary and secondary tumours.

Ependymoma, although rare, must not be overlooked. The development of compression symptoms should immediately alert the clinician to the potential seriousness of the situation, as spinal cord compression can have devastating and permanent consequences if not recognised and managed without delay.

It is also worth noting that back pain is one of the most common complaints in primary care, yet behind this common presentation may lie a serious, life-altering condition. Clinicians must therefore strike a careful balance between avoiding unnecessary investigations for benign causes and maintaining a high index of suspicion for more sinister pathology. This case demonstrates the dangers of complacency and the importance of not dismissing persistent, unexplained pain.

Case Study 11

Elevated MCV

The patient was a 60-year-old Caucasian woman who had been registered at our practice for 15 years. She was married and lived with her husband in a semi-detached house, leading a stable and content life. They had one grown-up daughter. She worked locally as a cleaner in nearby shops. She had never smoked, drank alcohol only socially and occasionally, and was otherwise in good health.

She attended the practice in the year 2000 for a routine follow-up of her blood pressure. She had a history of hypertension, monitored with yearly blood tests, particularly renal function and a full blood count. During this visit, she specifically asked if her liver function and thyroid function could also be checked, and I agreed to her request. The results showed all parameters within the normal range, except for her mean corpuscular volume (MCV), which was elevated at 103 fL.

I invited her to return to the surgery to review the situation and take a more detailed history. She reiterated that she was only an occasional social drinker, and there was nothing in her account to suggest excess alcohol intake. She reported no diarrhoea, abdominal pain, or malabsorption symptoms, and denied sensory loss or neurological complaints. Her appetite was preserved, her diet was balanced with regular consumption of meat and vegetables, and she had not experienced any weight loss.

On examination, she looked well, with no signs of anaemia, cyanosis, or systemic illness. Her temperature was 37.1°C, pulse 82 beats per minute, blood pressure 145/81 mmHg, weight 70 kilograms, and height 174 centimetres. Respiratory examination was unremarkable, and the cardiovascular system revealed no abnormalities beyond her mild hypertension. The abdomen was soft and non-tender, with no palpable hepatomegaly or splenomegaly, and there was no evidence of ascites, spider naevi, or lymphadenopathy. There was no flapping tremor.

A full neurological assessment, including cranial nerves, upper and lower limb reflexes, power, sensation, coordination, and plantar responses, was entirely normal. Peripheral circulation was intact.

To further investigate the raised MCV, repeat blood tests were arranged one week later, including vitamin B12, folate, and thyroid function. All of these came back normal. The patient was contacted and informed that no abnormality had been detected and that the isolated MCV elevation was difficult to explain. At this stage we agreed to careful observation, with reassurance that she should report any new symptoms such as tiredness, breathlessness, or easy bruising.

Her past medical history included hypertension, treated with amlodipine 5 mg and indapamide 2 mg daily, and a history of polymyalgia rheumatica, which had been treated with steroids two years earlier and had since resolved. She had no known allergies. Her medicines had been stable for some time, and there were no drugs on her list commonly associated with macrocytosis.

Key Questions

1. **What is the differential diagnosis, and which is the most likely one?**
2. **How would you manage this case?**

At this stage, the isolated raised MCV required careful interpretation. The main possibilities included thyroid disease, vitamin B12 deficiency, folate deficiency, alcohol excess, medication-related changes such as those seen with methotrexate, and blood disorders such as myelodysplasia.

Reticulocytosis, liver disease, and less common causes like aplastic processes can also elevate MCV. However, in this patient there was no supporting evidence clinically or biochemically for nutritional deficiency, thyroid disease, alcohol misuse, or drug effect, and her liver profile was normal.

I contacted the haematology department to discuss the case. Their advice was to monitor the situation by repeating her full blood count, vitamin B12, folate, gamma-GT, and thyroid function every three months. The rationale was straightforward: in the absence of symptoms or additional abnormalities, observation is often the safest and most informative strategy, allowing time to distinguish transient laboratory fluctuation from evolving disease.

For more than two years, this plan was followed carefully. Her MCV rose gradually to 106 fL, but she remained entirely well and asymptomatic, continued to work, and reported no fatigue, infections, bleeding, or weight loss. The haematology team continued to recommend observation, and she was reassured at each review, with clear safety-netting advice to return sooner if new symptoms developed.

After two years and three months, however, her blood count revealed new abnormalities, with evidence of anaemia. She also reported shortness of breath, which correlated with this finding and represented the first meaningful change in her clinical picture. At this stage I re-contacted the haematology department urgently. They arranged a bone marrow examination, which confirmed that she had developed myelodysplastic syndrome. Sadly, within six months of this diagnosis, her condition progressed to acute leukaemia, and despite best efforts, she passed away.

This case demonstrates the importance of vigilance in following up unexplained results. For more than two years, the only abnormality had been an elevated MCV, with no accompanying symptoms or abnormal findings. Eventually, the condition declared itself as a serious bone marrow disorder. The initial restraint – observing carefully while reversible causes were excluded – was appropriate; equally important was the prompt escalation once the full blood count changed and symptoms appeared.

Final Diagnosis

Myelodysplastic syndrome presenting with isolated macrocytosis, later progressing to acute leukaemia.

Comment

This case highlights the value of persistence and continuity in clinical medicine. A seemingly minor abnormality was in fact the earliest marker of a serious haematological disease. The case also shows the importance of open communication with patients, so that they understand why ongoing monitoring is required even in the absence of symptoms.

Finally, it underlines the reality that not every abnormality has an immediate explanation, and sometimes the passage of time is necessary for the true nature of a condition to become clear. The progression from unexplained macrocytosis to myelodysplasia, and eventually to acute leukaemia, illustrates the natural history of bone marrow failure syndromes and provides a powerful reminder of why vigilance is essential in general practice.

Lesson Learned

A raised MCV should never be dismissed, even when the patient feels entirely well and first-line tests are normal. Exclude common causes - B12 or folate deficiency, alcohol, thyroid disease, and drug effects - but be prepared to observe over time if nothing obvious is found. Clear follow-up intervals, consistent laboratory monitoring, and explicit advice about red-flag symptoms are essential. Persistent, isolated macrocytosis can be the earliest sign of myelodysplasia; if new symptoms or additional blood count changes emerge, urgent specialist reassessment is warranted.

Case Study 12

Low Mood and Unwell

This patient was a 62-year-old lady, originally from East Africa, who had been registered with the practice for many years along with her husband. They lived not far from the surgery. She was married with four grown-up children, two of whom lived nearby and the other two around London. She maintained close contact with her daughters, who were supportive and involved in her care. She had never smoked, did not drink alcohol, and had devoted much of her time to looking after her husband, who had suffered a stroke two years earlier. She was well known to the practice and had generally remained in stable health, apart from her history of hypertension.

She booked an appointment to see me, explaining on arrival that she was not feeling herself. She appeared subdued and low in mood, and reported that for the past twelve months she had been feeling increasingly unwell. This gradual decline was interfering with her ability to manage daily life and household responsibilities. For the first time, she had begun to rely on her daughters for help, which she found frustrating as she had always been independent and active in caring for her family.

She described loss of appetite and an unintentional weight loss of about three kilograms. Fatigue was becoming a major problem, to the extent that she was struggling to walk any distance without feeling exhausted. She denied cough, wheeze, diarrhoea, vomiting, or changes in her bowel habit. There was no history of chest pain. However, she admitted to mild but persistent back pain, mainly in the lower region. She had managed this discomfort with paracetamol and had thought little of it, regarding it as part of the normal ageing process. Recently, however, it had become more troublesome, although still without radiation.

Her past medical history included pneumonia ten years earlier and long-standing hypertension, well controlled with amlodipine 5 mg once daily. She had no known allergies. On examination, she looked slightly pale. Her temperature was 36.7°C, pulse 90 beats per minute in sinus rhythm, and blood pressure 125/72 mmHg. Cardiovascular assessment revealed normal heart sounds with no murmurs and no signs of heart failure. Chest expansion was good and breath sounds were vesicular without added sounds.

The abdomen was soft and non-tender, with the liver and spleen not palpable. There were a few small lymph nodes in the right iliac fossa, non-tender, each of them less than one centimetre in size. Examination of the back revealed a full range of movement, reflexes were preserved, and peripheral pulses were intact. Upper limbs and cranial nerves were unremarkable. Apart from her subdued mood, there were no abnormal neurological findings.

In discussion with her, we agreed to arrange a series of investigations. A full blood count, liver function tests, calcium, and a chest X-ray were requested. She returned one week later with the results. Her haemoglobin was 9 g/dL, showing normocytic, normochromic anaemia. The ESR was raised at 55. The remainder of the full blood count showed no significant abnormality. Renal function was normal with urea 6 and creatinine 100. Liver function tests were within normal limits, though the gamma globulin was slightly raised. The chest X-ray, arranged earlier, was normal.

At this stage, two important questions had to be asked.

Key Questions

1. **What is the differential diagnosis and what is the most likely diagnosis?**
2. **How do you manage this case?**

The presence of anaemia, raised ESR, fatigue, weight loss, and low mood prompted consideration of several possibilities. Tuberculosis was a possibility, particularly in view of her background and the raised ESR, but the normal chest X-ray and absence of respiratory symptoms argued against it. Carcinomatosis, whether primary or metastatic, might also cause weight loss and anaemia, but no masses or organ enlargement had been found.

Sepsis or bacterial endocarditis could also present with raised ESR and anaemia, yet her examination was entirely normal and she had no fever or cardiac signs. These alternatives seemed less convincing. The combination of normocytic, normochromic anaemia, raised ESR, raised gamma globulin, weight loss, and persistent back pain suggested a plasma cell disorder, most likely multiple myeloma.

In terms of management, the correct step was to seek specialist input urgently. Serum protein electrophoresis was therefore arranged and revealed a paraprotein band. With the suspicion strengthened, I contacted the haematology department at the local hospital, explained the case, and they arranged to see her without delay.

In hospital, further investigations were performed. A spinal X-ray revealed typical osteolytic lesions in the lower spine. Her calcium was raised, and bone marrow aspiration confirmed the diagnosis of multiple myeloma. She was commenced on treatment, but despite intensive therapy her disease progressed rapidly, and sadly she passed away four months later.

Final Diagnosis

Multiple myeloma presenting with anaemia, fatigue, weight loss, and back pain.

Comment

This case illustrates how multiple myeloma may present in an insidious manner, with vague and non-specific features. At first, her complaints of tiredness, weight loss, and low mood could easily have been dismissed as ageing, stress, or the burden of caring for her husband. The anaemia was not distinctive, being normocytic and normochromic, and might have been explained as anaemia of chronic disease. Her back pain was mild, controlled with paracetamol, and easily dismissed as degenerative.

However, when all the findings were brought together – anaemia, raised ESR, fatigue, weight loss, subtle back pain, and raised gamma globulin – the picture became concerning and pointed toward multiple myeloma. The case is a reminder of the need to integrate apparently minor details, rather than considering them in isolation. By linking the clues, the correct diagnosis can be reached.

Lesson Learned

The lesson learned from this case is that general practitioners must be cautious not to overlook the subtle presentations of serious disease. Multiple myeloma often develops slowly, and its early manifestations can appear deceptively benign. Careful correlation of symptoms and test results is crucial. Persistent unexplained anaemia, raised inflammatory markers, and chronic bone pain should always prompt further investigation, even when each finding alone seems non-specific. Early specialist referral is essential, as treatment outcomes are best when disease is recognised before complications such as fractures, renal impairment, or severe hypercalcaemia arise.

Case Study 13

Abdominal Pain and Temperature

The patient was a 60-year-old Irish gentleman who lived alone. His wife had left him about 18 months before he came to see me, although he had been registered in the practice for the past ten years.

He had always enjoyed his pint, but unfortunately his excessive drinking eventually led to the loss of his job. Dismissed almost a decade earlier, he never worked again and had been surviving on social security. He was a long-term smoker, averaging one pack of cigarettes a day. He had one son, now grown up and living in Scotland, but they had only occasional contact, and he largely managed his life in isolation.

He attended the practice complaining of abdominal pain, feeling unwell, and running a temperature for the past ten days. He denied cough, night sweats, diarrhoea, or vomiting. His history was marked by recurrent admissions to hospital with abdominal pain and jaundice, usually related to heavy drinking.

He would typically spend a week or ten days on the ward and then be discharged, only to reappear with similar problems later. Efforts to involve him in local alcohol support services were unsuccessful, as he repeatedly disengaged despite encouragement. Until this visit, however, he had not suffered from progressive weight loss, persistent oedema, or prolonged poor health. He had no known allergies and was not on regular medication, apart from occasional analgesia.

On this occasion he looked subdued and concerned. His temperature was 38.9°C, pulse 115 beats per minute, and blood pressure 120/69 mmHg. There were no cardiac murmurs or added sounds. His chest was clear with vesicular breath sounds, though there was an occasional wheeze from long-standing smoking. There were no clinical signs of pneumonia.

On abdominal examination, the spleen was palpable three fingerbreadths below the costal margin. The liver was enlarged, smooth, and extended four fingerbreadths below the costal margin, non-tender to palpation. Ascites was present, and there was a smooth, tender central abdominal mass. Both lower limbs showed pitting oedema. The overall picture suggested advanced liver disease with possible malignancy.

Key Questions

1. **What do you think might be wrong with this gentleman?**
2. **What is the action plan?**

The differential diagnosis at this stage had to be broad. His fever and abdominal findings could suggest intra-abdominal sepsis, such as a pyogenic abscess or even a tuberculous abscess. Given his background of alcoholism, alcoholic hepatitis or decompensated cirrhosis were strong considerations.

Long-term alcohol misuse also predisposes to hepatocellular carcinoma, particularly when associated with underlying viral hepatitis B or C, and this possibility had to be taken seriously. Other causes of abdominal masses, such as cholangiocarcinoma, secondary deposits from another primary, or even pancreatic carcinoma, also entered the differential. Carcinomatosis was a more remote possibility.

Taken together, the overall picture was one of significant hepatic disease, most likely malignant, though infection still had to be excluded.

In terms of management, the situation was well beyond the scope of primary care. A febrile patient with hepatomegaly, splenomegaly, ascites, oedema, and a central mass required urgent admission. I contacted the hospital, spoke to the medical registrar on call, dictated a referral letter, and arranged his immediate transfer.

Once admitted, he underwent full investigations including hepatitis serology, abdominal ultrasound, paracentesis for culture and cytology, and measurement of alpha-fetoprotein. A biopsy was also performed. The results confirmed hepatocellular carcinoma, supported by a raised alpha-fetoprotein level. Unfortunately, the tumour was advanced and no curative treatment was possible.

He was discharged under supportive care, but despite follow-up his health declined rapidly. Within four months he passed away.

Final Diagnosis

Advanced hepatocellular carcinoma on a background of alcohol-related liver disease.

Comment

This case illustrates the devastating course of long-term alcohol misuse, progressing through cirrhosis to hepatocellular carcinoma. For years his drinking had led to repeated admissions with abdominal pain and jaundice, but he always recovered enough to be discharged and resume his lifestyle.

The sudden appearance of hepatosplenomegaly, ascites, oedema, fever, and an abdominal mass signalled a turning point. At that stage, the differential was wide, including infective, inflammatory, and malignant causes, but the possibility of hepatocellular carcinoma stood out, and was later confirmed.

The case also shows the human cost of alcohol dependency, not only in terms of medical consequences but also in the way it isolates patients socially and emotionally. Despite contact with services, he was unable to engage meaningfully with alcohol support. His illness therefore progressed unchecked, culminating in a diagnosis that came too late for curative treatment.

Lesson Learned

The lesson learned is that in any patient with cirrhosis who deteriorates and develops ascites or an abdominal mass, malignancy must be suspected until proved otherwise. At the same time, infection should not be overlooked, especially in patients with poor nutrition and alcohol-related immunosuppression.

The role of the GP is limited to recognising the gravity of the presentation, initiating urgent referral, and ensuring prompt hospital involvement. Sadly, despite appropriate action, the diagnosis in this case came too late for curative treatment, and the outcome was poor. Early recognition of alcohol misuse and more sustained engagement with support services remain crucial preventive strategies, though difficult to achieve in practice.

Case Study 14

Unwell, Urine Frequency and Tired

The patient was a 39-year-old lady who had come to the United Kingdom six years earlier from Eastern Europe with her husband and their two children, then aged eight and ten. They were living in rented accommodation, and while her husband worked as a forklift driver, she supported the family as a cleaner. She did not smoke, she did not drink, and together they lived as a happy and settled family.

Her past history was significant for systemic lupus erythematosus, diagnosed before leaving her home country. She had been maintained on long-term low-dose steroids, taking 5 mg daily, and on arrival in the UK this was continued as a repeat prescription under regular review. She was well known in the practice as a pleasant and cheerful lady who usually presented with a smile.

One day she booked an appointment because she was feeling unwell. On arrival she did not look her usual self. She appeared a little subdued, perhaps because of her illness. She explained that for the past ten days she had felt unusually tired and lacking in energy, which had led her to ask for a sick note so that she could take time off work. She reported increased frequency of micturition but denied dysuria or visible haematuria. There was no cough, diarrhoea, vomiting, or breathlessness. She did not complain of weight loss, but her overall sense was of slowing down, fatigue, and lack of vitality.

On examination she did not look anaemic, and there was no shortness of breath at rest. There were no bruises or petechiae, and the facial rash she had from her lupus appeared unchanged. Her temperature was 37.1°C, pulse

90 beats per minute in sinus rhythm, and blood pressure 145/89 mmHg. Cardiovascular examination revealed no murmurs, no pericardial rub, and no signs of heart failure.

Her respiratory system was normal, with trachea central, chest clear, and vesicular breath sounds throughout, without evidence of effusion. Abdominal examination was also unremarkable, with no palpable liver or spleen, no lymphadenopathy, and no tenderness. Peripheral circulation was intact. She mentioned that her joints ached, but there was no swelling or effusion. Neurological examination was normal.

A urine test showed a few red blood cells and mild proteinuria. A full blood count and ESR were arranged. She returned the next day and the results showed an ESR of 50, with otherwise non-specific changes. A repeat urine test two days later again showed a few red cells and mild proteinuria, but the culture was sterile. Her background history was otherwise unremarkable apart from lupus. She was not allergic to any medication and continued only her prednisolone 5 mg daily.

Key Questions

1. **What is the most likely diagnosis?**
2. **What further management do you suggest?**

The differential diagnosis was wide. A flare-up of her systemic lupus erythematosus had to be considered, particularly in view of her joint pains and general malaise. Infection also had to be kept in mind, given her immunosuppressed state. Pyelonephritis or a urinary tract infection seemed less likely because her urine was persistently sterile, though she had haematuria and mild proteinuria. Sepsis and bacterial endocarditis were possibilities, but there were no murmurs, no signs of emboli, and her cultures were negative. Carcinomatosis was also entertained but appeared highly unlikely. Another important consideration, given her immunocompromised state and the repeated sterile pyuria, was tuberculosis.

With this uncertainty, the best course was hospital referral. I contacted the physicians and dermatologists, already aware of her lupus, and suggested urological input as well because of the urinary abnormalities. She was admitted for further investigation.

During her stay, her temperature rose to 38.2°C. Her steroid dose was increased, and she developed glycosuria, which was thought to be related to the higher steroid dose. Despite repeated cultures, the urine remained sterile on three separate occasions, although microscopic haematuria and proteinuria persisted. She began to deteriorate further, becoming more unwell and fatigued.

Because no clear diagnosis emerged, a case conference was held between the physicians, dermatologists, and urologists. They concluded that the most likely explanation was genitourinary tuberculosis and recommended starting empirical anti-tuberculous therapy. Treatment was commenced. Within weeks her temperature fell and her general condition improved. A few weeks later the urine culture confirmed the diagnosis, growing Mycobacterium tuberculosis sensitive to the standard three first-line drugs. She continued on treatment for six to nine months under joint care between the hospital and community services, and gradually returned to good health.

Final Diagnosis

Genitourinary tuberculosis in an immunosuppressed patient with lupus.

Comment

This case demonstrates the diagnostic difficulty faced when an immunosuppressed patient presents with vague symptoms. The possibilities initially were broad: a lupus flare, sepsis, bacterial endocarditis, urinary tract infection, or even malignancy. Yet the persistent sterile pyuria and proteinuria, together with her immunosuppressed state, were crucial clues pointing towards tuberculosis.

The case also underlines the importance of multidisciplinary care. No single specialty could have solved the puzzle in isolation; it was only after collaboration between physicians, dermatologists, and urologists that the correct working diagnosis was made. The decision to start empirical treatment before culture confirmation was not taken lightly but proved decisive, as the patient's rapid clinical improvement validated the approach.

Lesson Learned

The lesson learned is that in any patient with lupus or other forms of immune suppression, who presents with sterile pyuria and systemic features such as fever and malaise, tuberculosis must always be considered. Early referral to hospital is vital, as there is little a GP can do beyond initiating investigations and arranging specialist assessment. Empirical treatment in selected cases is not only justified but can be lifesaving, as illustrated here. The case highlights the need to keep an open mind, recognise the limitations of primary care, and involve secondary care promptly to prevent deterioration.

Case Study 15

Long-Standing Itching

The patient was a 60-year-old Caucasian lady, retired, who had previously worked as a cleaner until about a year earlier. She had lost her husband to lung cancer around the same time, a life event that had left her feeling emotionally fragile, but determined to live independently. She had been a heavy smoker in the past, but had since stopped. She did not drink alcohol and otherwise lived a healthy lifestyle. She had been a patient at the practice for the past five years.

She presented with a long history of itching, which she admitted had been troubling her for more than two years. She had tried various over-the-counter remedies without benefit. The itching had become so severe that it was interrupting her sleep, leaving her tired and irritable during the day. She also noticed that hot baths aggravated the problem. Apart from the pruritus, she had no diarrhoea, vomiting, or other gastrointestinal complaints.

Her past medical history included diet-controlled diabetes and hypothyroidism, for which she was taking thyroxine. She reported no significant allergies except to flucloxacillin. On examination, she was of average build, weighing around 70 kilograms and measuring 165 centimetres in height. She was comfortable at rest, not breathless, and not anaemic. Her pulse was 90 beats per minute in sinus rhythm, and her blood pressure was 140/85 mmHg. Cardiovascular examination was normal.

Respiratory system was clear, with vesicular breath sounds and no signs of consolidation or effusion. Abdominal examination revealed no ascites, no hepatomegaly, and no lymphadenopathy. There was no lower-limb oedema. Neurological and musculoskeletal examination was unremarkable. She was not jaundiced, but there were clear scratch marks, consistent with her history of nocturnal itching.

Key Questions

1. **What is the differential diagnosis, and what is the most likely cause?**
2. **What further management would you suggest?**

At this point the differential diagnosis was wide. Itching in the elderly may arise from iron deficiency anaemia, skin disorders such as eczema or scabies, endocrine causes including hypothyroidism, systemic illnesses such as chronic renal failure, or haematological conditions such as Hodgkin lymphoma and other reticuloses. Carcinomatosis was another possibility. Simple dry skin is also a common but often overlooked cause. With such a broad list, it was difficult to establish the exact reason for her symptoms.

Initial investigations were arranged, including full blood count, ESR, renal and liver function tests. The results showed a normal ESR, normal full blood count, and essentially normal liver function tests except for a slightly raised alkaline phosphatase, which at the time was not regarded as significant. On this basis, I advised her to increase skin hydration and prescribed cetirizine 10 mg once daily.

She returned later to report that the itching had not improved. A referral to the local dermatology department was made. Their assessment did not reveal any specific abnormality and their advice was simply to continue with moisturisers and antihistamines. She was discharged back to primary care, but the problem persisted.

Nearly a year later she returned, still complaining of severe itching. Examination again was normal, apart from multiple scratch marks across her body. Repeat investigations were arranged, including liver function tests, full blood count, and auto-antibody screening. This time her alkaline phosphatase was significantly raised and anti-mitochondrial antibodies were positive. Other liver parameters showed only mild disturbance, and clinically she remained non-jaundiced.

The presence of raised alkaline phosphatase with positive anti-mitochondrial antibodies suggested primary biliary cirrhosis. She was referred urgently to the gastroenterology department. Further investigations included ultrasound, MRCP imaging, and finally a liver biopsy, which confirmed the diagnosis of primary biliary cirrhosis. She was commenced on appropriate treatment and followed closely in secondary care.

Final Diagnosis

Primary biliary cirrhosis presenting with persistent pruritus.

Comment

This case highlights the importance of considering primary biliary cirrhosis in older patients who present with persistent pruritus. The condition often manifests with itching years before jaundice or other signs of liver dysfunction appear. It is easy to overlook, as the symptom can be attributed to dry skin or minor dermatological problems, and even specialist dermatology review may miss the diagnosis if liver function is not carefully considered.

The delay between initial presentation and diagnosis in this case shows how subtle biochemical abnormalities, such as a slightly raised alkaline phosphatase, can be disregarded if not put into context. The progression from non-specific itching to a clear autoimmune liver disease illustrates the importance of persistence in reassessment and not being falsely reassured by normal early findings.

Lesson Learned

The lesson learned is that persistent, unexplained pruritus, particularly in middle-aged or older women, warrants a thorough systemic evaluation. Basic blood tests including full blood count, ESR, renal function, and especially liver function should be performed early. A mildly raised alkaline phosphatase should never be ignored. Testing for anti-mitochondrial antibodies can provide the crucial clue, as in this case.

Another important point is not to be falsely reassured by a normal dermatological opinion. While skin conditions are common causes of itching, systemic causes, including primary biliary cirrhosis, chronic renal failure, and even malignancy, must always be considered. Persistent itching of several years' duration should be treated as a red flag, prompting repeated reassessment and referral when initial evaluations are inconclusive.

In summary, this case underlines the need for vigilance in patients with chronic pruritus. The differential is wide, but careful integration of the history, examination, and investigation results can prevent years of delay in reaching the correct diagnosis.

Case Study 16

Temperature and Sweating

A 59-year-old Caucasian man, well known to the practice for many years, was the landlord of a busy public house situated only a short distance, approximately five hundred yards, from the surgery. He was a familiar and cheerful figure, always appearing in good spirits and usually accompanied by his wife whenever he attended the practice. He had lived a settled family life, married for many years, with two grown-up children aged 35 and 38. Despite a lifestyle that was far from ideal, he considered himself to be happy and content.

His daily habits included smoking one packet of cigarettes, which he had done for over three decades, and drinking four pints of beer every day as part of his routine in managing the public house. Nevertheless, his jovial manner, constant smile, and positive attitude gave the impression of a man who was enjoying life without obvious health concerns.

During a spell of fine summer weather, on a weekend when the surgery was closed, this man suddenly became unwell. His illness began with the abrupt onset of a high temperature and profuse sweating, which persisted for about 24 hours. He did not develop any of the usual accompanying symptoms such as cough, runny nose, vomiting, or diarrhoea.

He assumed it was a minor viral illness and attempted to manage it himself by taking paracetamol, hoping to alleviate the fever and discomfort. However, as the weekend progressed, instead of improving, his condition deteriorated noticeably. His temperature continued to rise, and he became increasingly unwell, eventually developing episodes of confusion and hallucinations, which greatly alarmed his wife. Recognising that the illness was beyond self-care, the couple contacted the out-of-hours medical service.

The out-of-hours doctor visited him at home. On arrival, the patient was clearly unwell. His temperature was recorded at 39.6°C, his pulse rate was 115 beats per minute, and his blood pressure measured 150/90 mmHg. Oxygen saturation was reassuring at 98 per cent on room air. His mental state was affected, as he was hallucinating, though he showed no evidence of photophobia or neck stiffness, which might have raised concern for meningitis.

Physical examination revealed little to explain his illness. The throat and chest were clear, with no abnormal sounds on auscultation. The heart sounds were normal, with no added murmurs or signs suggestive of heart failure. He was clinically hydrated, and his abdomen was soft and non-tender, without evidence of organomegaly. Examination of both upper and lower limbs was unremarkable, and no rash or skin lesions were observed.

The patient's past medical history was relevant but not alarming. Three years earlier he had suffered an episode of lobar pneumonia, from which he had recovered fully, and in the previous three years he had also experienced two urinary tract infections. He was not taking any regular medications, had no known drug allergies, and there was nothing of significance in his family history.

Key Questions

1. **What is the differential diagnosis?**
2. **How would you manage this case?**

Given the sudden onset of high fever with systemic upset, the differential diagnosis was broad. Viral infection was a reasonable consideration, as was another urinary tract infection or a recurrence of pneumonia, particularly given his previous history. Meningitis or septicaemia needed to be considered in view of the high temperature, tachycardia, and the fact that he was hallucinating. However, there was no neck stiffness, photophobia, or rash, and the examination did not reveal a definite infective focus. Other possibilities such as endocarditis or occult abscess were conceivable but not strongly supported by the clinical findings at the time.

In such a situation, where the patient was clearly unwell with a high fever and altered mental state, yet without a clear diagnosis, the most appropriate management was immediate transfer to hospital for further investigations and monitoring. This was precisely the decision taken by the out-of-hours doctor, who promptly arranged an ambulance. The patient was admitted to the Accident and Emergency department of the local hospital, where he underwent further assessment.

On arrival at hospital, the findings were very similar to those recorded earlier by the attending doctor. His chest X-ray showed no abnormality, urine examination and culture were unremarkable, and initial blood cultures did not provide an explanation for the illness. Despite extensive assessment, the diagnosis remained uncertain. At this point, a particularly astute and thorough junior doctor decided to revisit the patient's history, asking in detail about past travel. This proved to be the crucial turning point in the case.

When questioned, the patient recalled that he had travelled to Africa two years earlier, spending time in an area known to be endemic for malaria. He had been entirely well since that trip and had not considered it relevant to his current illness. However, the travel history immediately raised the suspicion of malaria. A blood film was urgently requested, and the result confirmed the presence of Plasmodium vivax. With this diagnosis established, appropriate antimalarial treatment was commenced without delay.

The patient responded rapidly to treatment. Within 48 hours his fever subsided, the hallucinations resolved, and he regained his usual cheerful disposition. He remained in hospital for a short period for monitoring but was soon discharged home, where he resumed his normal life and activities.

Final Diagnosis

Malaria (Plasmodium vivax) presenting with fever, confusion, and hallucinations.

Comment

This case offers valuable lessons for clinical practice. Firstly, it demonstrates the absolute importance of obtaining a thorough travel history whenever a patient presents with fever of unknown origin. Even travel that occurred years earlier may remain relevant, as the relapsing nature of certain types of malaria means they can present long after the initial exposure.

Secondly, it highlights the fact that malaria should never be excluded solely on the basis of time elapsed since travel. Plasmodium vivax in particular has the capacity to remain dormant in the liver and re-emerge long after apparent recovery, sometimes years after exposure.

The case also illustrates the importance of maintaining a broad differential diagnosis when assessing a patient with fever, especially when the initial clinical examination does not provide clear localisation. While common conditions such as pneumonia, urinary tract infection, and viral illnesses should always be considered, clinicians must remain alert to less common but potentially serious possibilities. This is especially true in the context of an increasingly mobile population, where international travel is frequent and infectious diseases not typically encountered in the United Kingdom may still present in general practice or hospital settings.

Lesson Learned

The lesson learned is that while examination findings and investigations are vital, it is often the history - sometimes overlooked or considered irrelevant – that provides the decisive clue. The diagnostic breakthrough in this case came from a junior doctor who took the time to explore the patient's travel history in detail, demonstrating that careful history-taking remains at the heart of good medical practice.

The patient's recovery was rapid once the diagnosis was confirmed, and he was able to return to his family and his work in the public house with his usual good humour. This reinforces the principle that persistence, vigilance, and curiosity in clinical medicine can be just as valuable as advanced investigations in reaching a correct diagnosis.

Case Study 17

Shortness of Breath

This case was seen in the medical department of the hospital in 1983. The patient was a 40-year-old man who lived alone. He was unmarried, a non-smoker, and a non-drinker. He was socially isolated, keeping largely to himself, apart from occasional interaction with his next-door neighbour. Despite this, he described himself as content with his life and without major social concerns.

He presented to accident and emergency complaining of increasing shortness of breath over the past few weeks. The breathlessness had come on gradually and was worsening with time. He denied cough, wheezing, fever, sweats, or chest pain. There were no other significant symptoms to point to an obvious underlying illness.

His past medical history revealed that he had previously been diagnosed with a duodenal ulcer. Rather than taking prescribed medication, he had chosen to manage the condition himself. He explained that he had modified his diet, relying heavily on vegetables and fruit, but he cooked them thoroughly, rarely eating anything raw. He was not taking any prescribed medication and reported no allergies.

On examination he was alert, cooperative, and in good spirits. He was 178 centimetres tall and weighed approximately 65 kilograms, giving him a rather slim build. His temperature was 36.8°C, pulse 88 beats per minute, and blood pressure 115/80 mmHg. Cardiovascular examination revealed normal heart sounds without murmurs or rubs.

Respiratory examination showed the trachea centrally placed. There was dullness to percussion over the right side of the chest, with markedly reduced breath sounds. The left lung was clear with vesicular breathing and no added sounds. There was no chest pain and he was not sweating. Abdominal examination was normal, with no palpable liver, spleen, or masses. There was no lymphadenopathy. His upper and lower limbs showed normal coordination, power, sensation, and reflexes, with no evidence of muscle wasting or neurological deficit.

Routine blood investigations were arranged, including a full blood count, renal and liver function tests, and ESR. The haemoglobin was 11 g/dL with a normocytic, normochromic picture. ESR was 20 mm/hr, within the normal range. Kidney and liver function tests were also normal. A chest X-ray confirmed a right-sided pleural effusion.

Key Questions

1. **What do you think might be the problem?**
2. **How would you manage this case?**

The differential diagnosis of a pleural effusion is wide. It may be classified as either transudate or exudate. Transudates are commonly associated with conditions such as congestive cardiac failure, cirrhosis, or nephrotic syndrome. In this patient, there was no clinical or biochemical evidence of cardiac, hepatic, or renal disease, making these less likely. Exudates may result from pneumonia, tuberculosis, collagen vascular disease, or malignancy. None of these seemed immediately applicable based on his history and initial investigations, though they could not yet be excluded.

The next step was both diagnostic and therapeutic. Given his shortness of breath, a pleural tap was performed to relieve symptoms and to establish the nature of the effusion. To everyone's surprise, the aspirate revealed frank blood – a haemothorax. This unexpected finding prompted urgent further investigation.

At this stage, the consultant leading the case, who had a background in gastroenterology, recognised that the cause might not be malignant or infective. After careful review, the diagnosis was made: scurvy, caused by severe vitamin C deficiency.

The key to the diagnosis lay in his dietary history. Although he consumed large amounts of vegetables and fruit, he always cooked them thoroughly. Vitamin C is destroyed by heat, and without any raw fruit or fresh uncooked vegetables in his diet, he had become profoundly deficient. The deficiency had led to fragile blood vessels, predisposing him to spontaneous bleeding into the pleural cavity.

Treatment with vitamin C supplementation led to a gradual improvement in his health and resolution of the effusion. His breathlessness settled, and with continued dietary advice, his condition stabilised. Over time he regained confidence, and with reassurance, he came to understand the importance of diet in preventing such illnesses from recurring.

Final Diagnosis

Haemothorax due to scurvy (vitamin C deficiency).

This case illustrates a rare but important cause of pleural effusion. The initial presentation was indistinguishable from common conditions such as infection, tuberculosis, or malignancy. However, careful attention to the dietary history provided the crucial clue.

Scurvy is now uncommon in developed countries, but it can still occur in individuals with highly restricted or unbalanced diets. In this patient, his habit of cooking all fruits and vegetables destroyed their vitamin C content, leading to deficiency. The result was vascular fragility and haemothorax, an unusual but well-documented complication.

The case also highlights the importance of keeping an open mind when faced with atypical findings. The discovery of blood in the pleural space immediately raised concern for trauma or cancer, yet in this instance the explanation lay in something far more fundamental. It emphasises how a simple but thorough dietary history can be as decisive as any advanced investigation.

Lesson Learned

The lesson learned is that even in modern practice, nutritional deficiencies must not be overlooked, especially in socially isolated individuals or those who self-manage chronic conditions. A broad differential is always required for pleural effusion, but history-taking remains the most powerful diagnostic tool.

This case serves as a reminder that sometimes the simplest explanation, rooted in basic nutrition, can be the correct one. It also illustrates the value of considering rare conditions, particularly when common causes do not fit the clinical picture.

Case Study 18

Abdominal Pain and Diarrhoea

This was a 62-year-old Caucasian gentleman, retired. He had worked for a Building Society for many years and retired seven years earlier, partly due to health problems. Four years previously, he had undergone a renal transplant and had since been on long-term immunosuppressive therapy. He lived in a semi-detached private house with his wife, and they had two grown-up children. He never smoked, though he drank socially.

His past medical history also included hypertension, controlled with amlodipine 5 mg daily, and osteoarthritis of mild to moderate severity, managed with paracetamol. He had no known allergies.

He booked an appointment at the practice shortly after returning from a two-week cruise holiday. The trip included visits to several countries, with a three-day stay in Egypt. While abroad he developed abdominal pain and diarrhoea. The diarrhoea was offensive, containing mucus and streaks of blood, and accompanied by a foul smell. He saw a local doctor who prescribed Ciproxin, but this brought little benefit. The diarrhoea eventually settled, but the abdominal pain persisted and became his main complaint.

Initially the pain was central, but in the days leading up to his return to the UK it had localised to the right upper quadrant. He had also begun to feel hot, with mild night sweats, and his energy levels dropped noticeably. There was no vomiting. He returned to the UK about a week later and came to see me, as the abdominal pain was worsening steadily day by day.

On examination he did not appear anaemic and was not short of breath at rest. His temperature was 37.9°C, pulse 100 beats per minute, and blood pressure 135/80 mmHg. He weighed 75 kilograms and was 176 centimetres tall. Cardiovascular examination showed normal heart sounds with no evidence of heart failure.

Respiratory system was normal, with trachea central, chest expansion equal, and vesicular breath sounds without added sounds. Abdominal examination revealed mild tenderness in the upper abdomen, though the liver and spleen were not palpable. No lymphadenopathy was detected. Neurological and musculoskeletal systems were normal, with no abnormal findings.

Key Questions

1. **What is the most likely diagnosis and what differential diagnoses should be considered?**
2. **How would you manage this patient?**

The patient agreed to initial investigations. The results showed haemoglobin 12.9 g/dL, ESR 50 mm/hr, and a white blood cell count of 15,000, indicating leukocytosis. Liver function tests demonstrated a raised alkaline phosphatase, but the transaminases and bilirubin were within the normal range.

The differential diagnosis was wide. Given his recent travel and immunosuppressed state, an infective cause was most likely. Amoebiasis was a strong consideration, especially as it is endemic in Egypt and other developing countries, where transmission occurs through contaminated food and water. An amoebic liver abscess was therefore high on the list. Other possibilities included bacterial liver abscess, cholangitis, or even viral hepatitis.

Hepatitis, however, was less likely considering that his transaminases and bilirubin were normal. Typhoid fever was another possibility, but this typically presents with low, rather than high, white blood cell counts. Malignancy, such as primary liver cancer or metastasis, had also to be kept in mind, but the acute presentation and travel history made this less convincing.

Given his fever, leukocytosis, raised inflammatory markers, and localised abdominal tenderness, the case was clearly beyond the scope of primary care. I dictated a referral letter, spoke directly with the surgical registrar on call, and arranged urgent admission to hospital for further evaluation.

In hospital, further investigations were undertaken. These included blood cultures, serology for typhoid and amoebiasis, and abdominal ultrasound. Aspiration of the lesion was performed, and the results confirmed an amoebic liver abscess. It was judged likely to have been contracted during his stay in Egypt. He was treated with metronidazole and responded promptly, with rapid improvement in his symptoms. He was discharged home soon afterwards, much improved and able to return to normal life.

Final Diagnosis

Amoebic liver abscess following recent travel to Egypt.

Comment

This case illustrates the importance of linking a patient's illness to their recent travel history. In this man, a background of immunosuppression from renal transplantation increased the seriousness of his presentation, making him more vulnerable to infection and less able to mount an effective immune response. The key clue lay in his stay in Egypt, where amoebiasis is common.

The progression of central abdominal pain shifting to the right upper quadrant, combined with fever, leukocytosis, raised ESR, and elevated alkaline phosphatase, made an infective liver abscess the most likely diagnosis. The ultimate confirmation by aspiration highlighted the value of combining clinical suspicion with targeted investigation.

Lesson Learned

The lesson learned is that recent travel history should always be sought in patients with abdominal or systemic illness, particularly when they have visited developing countries. Amoebiasis remains a significant global health issue, readily contracted through contaminated food and water, and can lead to life-threatening complications such as liver abscess.

This case also demonstrates the limits of primary care. While initial investigations can provide important information, urgent hospital referral is essential when serious infective or surgical conditions are suspected. In such cases, imaging, serology, and aspiration are required to establish the diagnosis and guide treatment.

Finally, the case underlines the importance of vigilance when caring for immunosuppressed patients, such as those who have undergone organ transplantation. Their presentations may be atypical, and infections that are uncommon in the general population may cause severe disease. Timely recognition and referral allowed this patient to make a full recovery.

Case Study 19

Post Appendicectomy Complication

The patient was a 17-year-old boy in the middle of his A Level studies. He was a bright, cheerful, and previously healthy young man who lived with his parents and three sisters in a close-knit family. He did not smoke or drink alcohol, and apart from the usual childhood illnesses of measles and gastroenteritis, he had never suffered from any medical problems.

In 1973, during my first houseman post, he was admitted via casualty to the medical ward where I was working. His history revealed that he had undergone an appendicectomy five weeks earlier. He had remained on the surgical ward for about a week and had been discharged once considered fit. At the time of discharge, however, he had already mentioned to the staff that he was troubled by suprapubic pain and discomfort in the lower back. He was reassured that this was normal after surgery and that simple painkillers such as paracetamol would suffice.

Once home, the discomfort persisted. The pain, initially localised to the suprapubic region, extended gradually to the coccygeal and perianal area. At first, he managed with occasional analgesia, but as the days went on the pain intensified, reaching the point where he could no longer tolerate it. He denied vomiting or diarrhoea, though he noticed that the pain eased slightly after passing stool. In time, he also developed night sweats. He did not complain of weight loss or urinary symptoms, and apart from the increasing pain he remained otherwise stable.

When I examined him, he looked unwell and in obvious discomfort. His pulse was 110 beats per minute, his temperature 38.5°C, and his blood pressure 110/70 mmHg. He did not appear anaemic. The heart sounds and chest were clear. His abdomen showed a healthy surgical scar and only mild suprapubic tenderness. The liver and spleen were not palpable, and the back appeared normal. Inspection of the perianal region revealed no haemorrhoids or external signs of disease. The neurological system was sound. At that time, no per rectum examination was performed, which was a critical omission.

Routine investigations revealed a raised white cell count of 17,000 and an ESR of 45, while renal and liver functions were normal. The working diagnosis was a post-operative infection. Following this reasoning, we prescribed Septrin, a broad-spectrum antibiotic widely used at the time, for a full week. Despite this, there was no improvement. His fever persisted, and his blood tests continued to show marked leukocytosis. His pain also intensified, adding to the concern that the diagnosis had not been fully established.

Key Questions

1. **What is the most likely diagnosis, and what are the possible differential diagnoses?**
2. **How should this case be managed?**

At this stage, the surgical team was asked to review him. The consultant surgeon examined the patient and, crucially, carried out a per rectum examination. With that, the diagnosis became immediately clear: a rectal abscess. He was promptly transferred back to the surgical ward, where incision and drainage were performed. The effect was dramatic. The fever settled, the blood count returned to normal, and the boy's pain quickly resolved. His recovery thereafter was smooth, and within a short time he was discharged home, able to resume his studies.

Final Diagnosis

Rectal abscess following appendicectomy.

Comment

This case carries several important messages. First, no clinical examination is complete without considering a per rectum assessment when pelvic or perineal symptoms are present. By failing to do this, we missed a straightforward diagnosis and delayed the correct treatment. Second, a persistently raised temperature and white cell count after surgery must always raise suspicion of an undrained source of infection. In such circumstances, antibiotics alone will never suffice: the focus of infection must be found and treated.

The patient himself had repeatedly complained of perineal pain, and this was a clear clue to the underlying problem. His words should have guided us more carefully, reminding us of the importance of listening to the patient's account as closely as we examine their body.

This experience also taught me, as a junior doctor, the importance of humility, reflection, and knowing when to seek help from senior colleagues. The surgical consultant's simple but thorough approach corrected our mistake and turned the case around.

Lesson Learned

The lesson learned is that diagnosis must always come before treatment. A comprehensive examination, including rectal examination where indicated, remains a cornerstone of safe clinical practice. Persistent fever and leukocytosis after surgery should immediately raise suspicion of a hidden source of infection, and treatment must address that source rather than rely solely on antibiotics.

Finally, this case reinforced a truth that has guided me throughout my career: medicine is not just about knowledge or technology, but about careful listening, thorough examination, and the courage to admit when we need help. This young man made a full recovery, but the lessons he left with us as doctors were enduring and invaluable.

Case Study 20

Shortness of Breath

This lady had been seen in the practice for many years. She was a 44-year-old woman at the time, married with two children, boys aged ten and 12. She worked as a receptionist at a solicitor's office for several years. She had never smoked, was only a social drinker, and lived in a bungalow with her husband and children, enjoying a happy and stable family life. She was well-known to us as a reliable patient who usually came for routine reviews, rather than urgent problems.

In the year 2000, she came to see me with a history of shortness of breath that had been troubling her for the previous two weeks. In fact, the story went back nearly two years, when she had suffered a pulmonary embolism. She had been admitted to the local hospital, treated with warfarin, and had since been maintained on a daily dose of 4 mg. She was attending the anticoagulation clinic regularly, and her INR was consistently within the therapeutic range. She had adjusted well to the long-term medication and had not required additional treatment until now.

She explained that her current breathlessness had first been noticeable on exertion, such as climbing stairs or walking briskly, but it was gradually worsening. She found it increasingly difficult to climb even a single flight of stairs without stopping to rest. She had no cough, coryza, or wheeze. She denied chest pain, palpitations, or hemoptysis. There was no swelling of the legs, calf tenderness, or history of recent surgery. She was not on contraceptives, and there was no family history of clotting disorders.

The patient had attended Accident and Emergency a few days earlier, but no abnormality had been found and she was discharged home. Four days later she returned to the practice, saying she was deteriorating. Her words were striking: 'I can't go on anymore. There must be something wrong. I wonder if you can help me.' This persistence and her obvious distress reinforced the need for urgent re-evaluation.

Her past medical history was significant only for pulmonary embolism. She had no allergies and continued warfarin regularly. On examination she was not anaemic, and there was no cyanosis, but she was clearly short of breath, even at rest. Her respiratory rate was 22 per minute. Her pulse was 98 beats per minute, regular, in sinus rhythm. Blood pressure was 125/75 mmHg. The heart sounds were normal with no murmurs or added sounds. Chest examination revealed a central trachea, vesicular breath sounds bilaterally, no signs of pneumothorax, no pleural rub, and no added sounds such as wheeze or crepitations. Oxygen saturation on room air was 95 per cent. Both upper and lower limbs were unremarkable, with no evidence of DVT. Importantly, a D-dimer had not been carried out during her previous hospital attendance.

Previous investigations had included a chest X-ray, which was normal, and routine blood tests, which were also normal. Haemoglobin was 13.1 g/dL, white cell count 8,000, and there was no eosinophilia. ESR was normal. Liver function showed only minimal disturbance, with LDH and transaminases marginally raised, while renal function remained normal. These findings offered no obvious explanation for her worsening breathlessness.

Key Questions

1. **What do you think the differential diagnosis is?**
2. **How would you manage her?**
3. **What do you think the final diagnosis was?**

Clearly, she was short of breath, yet clinical examination failed to reveal a definite cause. Several possibilities were considered. First, it could have been a primary chest problem such as recurrent pulmonary embolism or early interstitial lung disease, though there were no physical signs. A second possibility was a cardiac problem, particularly pulmonary hypertension or right-sided strain, which might not be detected on examination alone. A third possibility was anxiety with hyperventilation, though her persistence, deterioration, and lack of previous psychiatric history made this less likely.

At this stage, further investigations were essential. She required an echocardiogram to exclude cardiac causes, particularly right heart strain, and ideally a CT pulmonary angiogram to look for fresh emboli, although this was not readily available in 2000. A ventilation-perfusion scan was considered the most appropriate next step. In primary care, we did not have access to D-dimer testing, which could have provided supportive evidence. Recognising the urgency, I contacted the radiology department, explained the situation, and requested an urgent ventilation-perfusion scan. They agreed, and she was seen promptly.

Final Diagnosis

Recurrent small pulmonary emboli.

Comment

This case was both challenging and instructive. The key lesson was to take the patient's history seriously. She knew something was wrong and pressed for help. Despite being on warfarin with therapeutic INR levels, she had nevertheless developed further pulmonary emboli. It is crucial to recognise that anticoagulation reduces risk but does not eliminate it entirely. The absence of calf swelling or signs of deep vein thrombosis did not rule out pulmonary embolism, and her presentation demonstrated how emboli can recur in a subtle but dangerous way.

The case also highlighted the importance of persistence. The patient persisted in seeking help because she recognised her condition was deteriorating. As her GP, I persisted in pursuing further investigations despite normal examination and blood results. Without this, her recurrent emboli might have been missed until catastrophic complications occurred.

Finally, this case underlined the value of continuity of care in general practice. Because I had known her for years, I could recognise the change in her usual health and respond appropriately. That personal knowledge, combined with listening carefully and acting promptly, ensured the correct diagnosis was reached and treatment could be initiated without delay.

Case Study 21

Temperature and Anaemia

A 57-year-old man had joined the practice 12 months earlier. He was married and lived with his wife in a bungalow. He had never smoked and drank wine occasionally. His main care had long been under the QE Hospital, where he was followed regularly after a heart transplant. His visits to the practice were mostly for repeat prescriptions issued by the hospital, along with occasional minor concerns.

He presented with a history of fever for one week, for which he had been taking paracetamol without improvement. He reported no cough, coryza, vomiting, diarrhoea, abdominal pain, dysuria, or haematuria. The QE Hospital had already performed baseline investigations. His full blood count showed haemoglobin of 10 g/dL with normochromic, normocytic anaemia, and a white cell count of 10,000/μL. Liver function tests were normal. Urinalysis was negative for protein and blood, and culture showed no growth. Renal function was also normal.

On Friday evening, he attended the practice again, requesting review. He reported losing one stone in weight during the preceding month, accompanied by persistent fever. On examination, his weight was 78 kilograms, height 180 centimetres, blood pressure 140/79 mmHg, pulse 100 beats per minute, and temperature 38°C. The throat was unremarkable. In the groin, two mobile and tender lymph nodes about 1 centimetre in size were noted, and in the right posterior cervical triangle there were a couple of soft, non-tender nodes of similar size.

The patient's chest expansion was normal, with no added sounds, crepitations, or signs of consolidation or effusion. Vesicular breath sounds were preserved. Jugular venous pressure was normal, and heart sounds were normal with no added sounds. Abdominal examination revealed hepatomegaly, 3 centimetres below the costal margin, and splenomegaly, also 3 centimetres below the costal margin, both smooth and non-tender. There were no signs of ascites. The limbs showed no ulceration, and peripheral circulation was intact. Neurological examination was grossly normal.

At this stage the differential diagnosis was wide. Possible causes included infective conditions such as viral or pyogenic infections and tuberculosis, collagen disorders, and malignant disease such as carcinomatosis. The purpose here is not to provide a comprehensive list of all causes of fever but to highlight the breadth of possibilities. For instance, urine should be examined for haematuria in suspected hypernephroma, or tested for pyogenic infection and tuberculosis. Chest X-ray is valuable to exclude empyema or abscesses. At this stage, the most likely diagnosis was difficult to pinpoint, but given the patient's immunosuppressed state, an infective cause remained a major concern.

How could the diagnosis be established? Unfortunately, time could not be wasted. Securing an early diagnosis was vital and might even be life-saving. The earlier it was achieved, the better the chance of survival. At this stage, I advocated proceeding with a biopsy of the liver or enlarged lymph nodes. Such tissue examination could reveal tuberculosis, pyogenic infection, or carcinomatosis, among others. In the 1980s, when this case occurred, MRI and CT scanning were not widely available, so histology was often the most decisive approach.

The hospital letter documented repeated urine and sputum cultures, all negative, as well as an inconclusive chest X-ray that showed minor changes but no firm evidence of infection, consolidation, or lymphadenopathy. Despite conservative measures, the patient's condition deteriorated, with persistently high temperatures and drenching sweats. In view of his immunosuppressed state and progressive decline, the team at the QE Hospital decided to proceed with a liver biopsy, which yielded the diagnosis.

Final Diagnosis

Tuberculosis of the liver.

Comment

This case illustrates the considerable diagnostic challenge of persistent pyrexia in an immunosuppressed patient with a history of cardiac transplantation. The broad differential diagnosis included bacterial infections such as endocarditis or intra-abdominal abscess, malignancies such as lymphoma or leukaemia, granulomatous conditions such as sarcoidosis, and a range of viral, fungal, and protozoal infections.

Despite repeated investigations, no causative organism or clear pathology was identified. The presence of hepatosplenomegaly and lymphadenopathy widened the spectrum of possibilities. Imaging, including chest X-ray, was inconclusive. Ultimately, a tissue diagnosis was essential, and the liver biopsy provided the answer.

Lesson Learned

In immunosuppressed patients with unexplained fever, tuberculosis must always be considered, even when there is no pulmonary involvement. Modern imaging such as CT and MRI may suggest hepatic or nodal lesions, but biopsy remains the gold standard for confirmation and for guiding treatment. Early escalation to tissue diagnosis can be life-saving, as delays in reaching a diagnosis may compromise outcome. Even with appropriate diagnosis and treatment, immunosuppression presents a major barrier to recovery, highlighting the importance of rapid identification and targeted management.

Case Study 22

Bowel Obstruction

This was a patient known to the practice for more than ten years, who regularly attended with his family. He was a 24-year-old plumber, a non-smoker, but a regular drinker, consuming around four pints a day, sometimes more at weekends. Despite this, he was well-behaved, a reliable young man, living with his parents and working continuously without interruption.

This young man eventually presented with abdominal pain that progressed to bowel obstruction, requiring surgical intervention. Looking back, I had seen him 12 months earlier with abdominal pain. He described central abdominal discomfort that came and went, not associated with vomiting or diarrhoea. The pain was episodic, disappearing and returning without a clear pattern. He had never noticed blood in his stools.

On examination at that time, he appeared well nourished, active, and cheerful. His weight was 75 kilograms and his height 178 centimetres. His pulse was 80 beats per minute and blood pressure 120/80 mmHg. The abdomen was soft, with no tenderness, no masses, and no organomegaly; the liver was not palpable. Bowel sounds were normal. Cardiovascular and respiratory examinations were also unremarkable. In view of these findings, he was reassured.

At the first consultation he was prescribed a simple painkiller, which did not provide lasting relief. He re-attended a couple of weeks later with the same complaint. Re-examination was again unremarkable, and his observations remained stable.

Key Questions

1. What is the differential diagnosis?
2. How would you manage this case?
3. What was the final diagnosis?

At that stage, further investigations were requested, including full blood count, renal function, electrolytes, calcium, and liver function tests. The haemoglobin was 12.5 g/dl with normal indices, there was no leukocytosis, ESR was 10, and renal and liver profiles were within normal limits. Calcium was also normal. With no abnormal findings, the impression was possible irritable bowel syndrome, and antispasmodics were prescribed. These gave only temporary relief, after which he stopped attending the surgery regularly.

Instead, he presented on several occasions to the Accident and Emergency department. The same impression was reached there, and once again basic investigations were repeated with unremarkable results. He was discharged with painkillers each time, until eventually the situation escalated.

Repeated attendance is always a red flag. A young, working man, with no psychological overlay and a consistent story, should have prompted earlier escalation beyond basic blood tests. Irritable bowel syndrome was initially considered, but this condition cannot explain obstruction and should remain a diagnosis of exclusion. Renal colic was unlikely with normal calcium and no blood in the urine.

Appendicitis did not fit the prolonged, episodic course and would not account for multiple attendances over the year. Infective causes such as intra-abdominal abscess were improbable in the absence of fever or leukocytosis. Pancreatitis was thought of because of his drinking habits, yet serum amylase remained normal.

At that stage, further imaging should have been pursued. Early use of ultrasound or MRI could have helped in identifying structural disease such as Crohn's disease or another inflammatory bowel condition. Endoscopic assessment or contrast studies might also have been considered if symptoms persisted despite normal routine investigations.

Ultimately, after yet another emergency presentation, he was referred to the surgical team. CT and MRI scans were undertaken, which revealed small bowel narrowing. At laparotomy, he was diagnosed with Crohn's disease causing obstruction due to stricture formation. The operation confirmed the underlying pathology that had eluded detection during his repeated earlier attendances.

Final Diagnosis

Crohn's disease.

Comment

This case highlights how easily chronic inflammatory bowel disease can be missed in young patients when the presentation is vague and intermittent. Abdominal pain that comes and goes, in the absence of abnormal blood tests, is often attributed to functional causes such as irritable bowel syndrome. However, IBS is a diagnosis of exclusion and should never be assumed in the face of persistent or worsening symptoms.

In this young man, repeated attendances both in primary care and emergency departments should have triggered earlier escalation to imaging or endoscopy. His eventual diagnosis of Crohn's disease was only made at laparotomy when obstruction occurred, by which time the disease had progressed significantly.

Lesson Learned

Repeated presentations are a warning sign and must not be overlooked. Patients who attend both primary care and hospital services again and again, particularly young working individuals who are not in the habit of seeking medical attention unnecessarily, should be investigated more thoroughly. Irritable bowel syndrome is a diagnosis of exclusion and should never be assumed without ruling out organic causes, especially in persistent or recurrent abdominal pain.

Early imaging is crucial. When routine blood tests are normal but abdominal pain recurs, investigations such as ultrasound, CT, or MRI may reveal the underlying pathology. Inflammatory bowel disease should always be kept in mind, as delayed diagnosis carries the risk of severe complications, including obstruction, perforation, and the need for major surgery.

Case Study 23

Abdominal Pain

This case was seen in the medical department in 1980, The patient was a 37-year-old Afro-Caribbean lady, single, with a 17-year-old son. She worked as a call handler for RCA and lived with her son in a semi-detached council house. She never smoked and drank alcohol only socially.

She had been attending the clinic with abdominal pain and persistently positive faecal occult blood tests. At that time, I had just started my role as a medical registrar, assisting a consultant whose outpatient list was fully booked.

The patient's history revealed intermittent, episodic abdominal pain over roughly twelve months. The pain was central, not related to her menstrual cycle, and without radiation to the back, upper and lower abdomen. Each episode could last a few days and then settle for weeks before recurring. She reported no weight loss, no change in bowel habit, no diarrhoea or mucus, and no rectal bleeding. She denied nausea and vomiting.

There was no haematuria, her periods were regular, and eating did not influence the pain. She had found that simple analgesia gave little benefit, and there were no clear triggers such as exertion, meals, or stress; the attacks seemed to come 'out of the blue,' then remit.

Her past medical history included an appendicectomy as a 12-year-old, with full recovery. She had mild asthma for which she used a salbutamol inhaler intermittently, and she was allergic to trimethoprim.

On assessment the patient was pleasant and cooperative, though understandably weary after repeated attendances without progress. She was not clinically anaemic. Height 176 centimetres, weight 70 kilograms.

Blood pressure 145/82 mmHg, pulse 70 beats per minute in sinus rhythm, temperature 37.2°C. Cardiovascular examination was normal with intact peripheral pulses. The chest was clear. Neurological examination (cranial nerves, power, tone and sensation) was normal. There were no abnormal abdominal findings at that stage. There was no clubbing, no peripheral oedema, and no perianal disease visible, and abdominal palpation revealed no masses or organomegaly; bowel sounds were normal.

As this was her first visit to me, I repeated the faecal occult blood and arranged routine tests including a full blood count, urea and electrolytes, liver function tests, and blood sugar. Results showed haemoglobin 11 g/dL with microcytosis (MCV 72), ESR 32 mm/hr, urea 7 mmol/L, creatinine 100 μmol/L, normal electrolytes, and normal liver enzymes including alkaline phosphatase.

The salient abnormalities were a microcytic anaemia with persistently positive faecal occult blood, suggesting ongoing blood loss without an obvious source. Iron studies would ordinarily be expected to confirm iron deficiency in this setting, but the immediate priority was to locate the bleeding site.

The patient returned to clinic two weeks later.

Key Questions

1. **What is the differential diagnosis?**
2. **How should the case be managed?**
3. **What is the final diagnosis?**

The central problem was clear: chronic, unexplained abdominal pain with microcytic anaemia and persistent faecal occult blood positivity. The first duty was to exclude carcinoma of the colon. Even without rectal bleeding, altered bowel habit, or weight loss, colonic cancer may present subtly in its early stages, and microcytosis is often a red flag for iron deficiency anaemia secondary to chronic blood loss.

Inflammatory bowel disease also had to be considered. Ulcerative colitis seemed less likely, as there was no diarrhoea, mucus, or tenesmus, yet it could not be completely ruled out. Crohn's disease, by contrast, was a stronger possibility, since it can present with intermittent abdominal pain, occult bleeding, and iron deficiency anaemia without obvious bowel habit changes. The episodic nature of her pain, with long symptom-free intervals, further supported this line of thought. Small-bowel involvement in Crohn's frequently escapes routine colonoscopy and can therefore present as 'occult' blood loss with iron deficiency and non-specific abdominal discomfort.

Other possibilities included haemorrhoids and anal fissures, though these would not explain the abdominal pain and would not persistently cause occult blood positivity between menstrual cycles. Menstrual contamination itself was a potential source of false positive results, but the consistent positivity in between periods argued strongly against this. Small-bowel pathology also had to be considered.

Polyps, angiodysplasia, or vascular malformations can cause occult bleeding and anaemia, but rarely present with pain of this character. Peptic ulcer disease was not suggested by the patient's history, as she had no dyspepsia, epigastric tenderness, or meal-related symptoms. Likewise, biliary and pancreatic causes were not supported by the absence of right upper quadrant tenderness, jaundice, or back-radiating pain.

After reviewing these possibilities, the working plan was clear. Following discussion with my consultant and a newly-appointed gastrointestinal surgeon, the consensus was to exclude colonic carcinoma first. In that era, careful stepwise investigation – rather than immediate advanced imaging – was the norm.

The patient underwent colonoscopy, which revealed no evidence of carcinoma and no features of ulcerative colitis. With colonic disease excluded, the focus shifted to the small bowel. A barium follow-through was arranged, which demonstrated the classical 'string sign,' strongly suggestive of Crohn's disease affecting the terminal ileum. The radiologist's report commented on segmental narrowing with proximal dilatation – findings which aligned with her intermittent colicky episodes and chronic iron deficiency.

Thereafter, the surgical and medical teams jointly assumed her care and commenced appropriate long-term management for Crohn's disease. For the patient, finally arriving at a unifying diagnosis brought relief after twelve months of uncertainty and repeated inconclusive testing. Education about disease course, nutritional support (including iron replacement), and a plan for medical therapy were instituted, with surgery reserved for complications.

Final Diagnosis

Crohn's Disease.

Lesson Learned

This case underscores the importance of never dismissing a persistently positive faecal occult blood test, particularly when accompanied by microcytic anaemia. Even in the absence of overt bleeding, weight loss, or altered bowel habit, the possibility of serious gastrointestinal disease must remain at the forefront. Carcinoma of the colon must always be excluded as a priority, for an early-stage malignancy can present without obvious warning signs. Once this is ruled out, clinicians must look beyond the colon and investigate the small bowel.

The case also highlights the importance of broad differential thinking. Ulcerative colitis and Crohn's disease often overlap in their presentations, but Crohn's disease can appear with subtle and intermittent symptoms, such as episodic abdominal pain and occult blood loss without diarrhoea. Small-bowel investigations, such as barium follow-through in this era, played a decisive role, and the finding of the string sign was virtually pathognomonic. Interpreting the anaemia as iron deficiency secondary to chronic blood loss helped to link the laboratory pattern with the radiology and the patient's symptoms.

False positive faecal occult blood tests should always be considered. Haemorrhoids, anal fissures, and menstrual contamination can all mislead, but they rarely account for the whole picture when other clinical features point elsewhere. The key is to interpret test results in the context of the patient's story, not in isolation. Equally important is the collaborative nature of good medicine. In this case, the coordinated input of both medical and surgical teams brought clarity after months of uncertainty. For the patient, the relief of finally knowing the cause of her symptoms was as important as the treatment itself.

Ultimately, the lesson is that persistence in investigation, careful exclusion of false positives, and multidisciplinary collaboration are the cornerstones of accurate diagnosis and good clinical care.

Case Study 24

Poorly-Controlled BP

A gentleman, 46 years old, who had recently moved from the north of England to the Midlands, came to register as a new patient at our practice. He had resettled with his wife and two children, aged 12 and 14, after securing employment with an insurance company. He described himself as generally well and enjoying family life. He never smoked and, apart from an occasional social drink, he did not drink alcohol regularly. He appeared content, sociable, and eager to establish good continuity of care with his new GP after leaving his long-term practice.

He attended the surgery for a new patient check-up, but during the consultation explained that his main problem was longstanding high blood pressure. His previous practice had struggled to achieve adequate control despite regular medication.

His past medical history included an appendicectomy at the age of ten, with no subsequent issues. He also had dry skin, for which he used moisturiser, and a melanoma excised from his left arm ten years earlier. He had been discharged from dermatology follow-up with reassurance that he was cancer-free. His only allergy was to dust, which caused sneezing and occasional nasal discharge.

At the time of registration, his medication consisted of bendroflumethiazide 2.5 mg once daily and olmesartan 40 mg once daily. On examination, he was a pleasant, well-presented man. His height was 180 centimetres and his weight 80 kilograms. Temperature was normal, and his pulse was 77 beats per minute in sinus rhythm, with a blood pressure of 160/92 mmHg.

Cardiac auscultation revealed no added sounds, and there were no signs of cardiac enlargement or failure. His respiratory and neurological examinations were normal, including fundoscopy, which showed no changes to suggest hypertensive damage. The limbs were symmetrical, reflexes intact, and peripheral circulation normal. Overall, he looked healthy, but his uncontrolled hypertension was of concern.

Because of the persistently high reading, I arranged a review one week later. A full set of blood tests was requested, including complete blood count, renal and liver function, cholesterol profile, fasting glucose, and HbA1c. When he returned, his blood pressure was again raised at 159/93 mmHg.

The investigations were mostly within normal limits, but his potassium was 3.2 mmol/L, slightly below the accepted range. His renal function was otherwise normal, with urea 5, creatinine 90, sodium 140, and liver tests unremarkable. Lipid profile and blood sugar were also satisfactory. The persistently low potassium stood out as the only abnormality, raising a flag for further exploration.

We discussed the result, and he explained that his previous GP had repeatedly noted potassium levels around 3.1 to 3.2 mmol/L. He had been told it was not significant, particularly as he had no symptoms. At this stage, I considered his diuretic therapy as a possible cause and decided to repeat the potassium after one month. Meanwhile, I awaited his medical records from his previous surgery. I explained to him that although he felt well, low potassium in the context of high blood pressure might suggest something more significant than a side effect of medication.

At his next visit, the potassium remained low at 3.1 mmol/L. By then his records had arrived, confirming persistently low potassium readings for several years. I explored possible explanations with him, asking about gastrointestinal upset such as diarrhoea or vomiting, but he denied these. He also had no history of laxative abuse or excessive liquorice consumption, both of which can rarely lead to hypokalaemia.

I explained that potassium loss could occur through the gut or the kidneys and that medications such as diuretics often played a role. Since his potassium had remained low despite good overall health, I suggested stopping bendroflumethiazide and replacing it with a calcium channel blocker. We agreed to start amlodipine 5 mg daily, with review in one month. Reviewed after a month, unfortunately the blood pressure was still the same, with no change, and the potassium level continued to linger between 3.1 and 3.2 mmol/L.

This persistence of hypokalaemia, even after stopping the diuretic, strongly suggested an alternative cause. His blood pressure remained high, indicating an underlying pathology beyond 'essential' hypertension. His presentation was in fact quite classical: hypertension plus hypokalaemia, in the absence of renal impairment or gastrointestinal potassium loss.

Key Questions

1. **What is the most likely explanation for his persistent hypokalaemia?**
2. **How would you manage this case?**

I referred him to the endocrinology clinic, and after a discussion with the consultant it was agreed he should undergo further investigation. The endocrinologist performed detailed hormonal studies, including plasma aldosterone and renin levels, and arranged imaging. The results showed an elevated aldosterone-to-renin ratio, consistent with primary hyperaldosteronism.

A CT/MRI scan revealed a left renal cortical adenoma. The diagnosis of primary hyperaldosteronism due to an adrenal adenoma was confirmed. He was referred to a surgeon, who discussed management with him, and subsequently the adenoma was resected. After the operation, his potassium returned to normal, but he was advised that blood pressure control might still require long-term monitoring and medication.

Final Diagnosis

Conn's syndrome (primary hyperaldosteronism due to adrenal adenoma).

This case highlights the importance of pursuing unexplained biochemical abnormalities in the context of hypertension. Although diuretics are a frequent cause of hypokalaemia, persistence of low potassium after withdrawal should raise suspicion of other causes of hyperaldosteronism. Adrenal hyperplasia or adenoma are classic conditions which can present with this pattern. In this man, the years of low potassium levels had been overlooked as clinically insignificant, but in fact they held the clue to the true diagnosis. Once identified and treated surgically, his prognosis improved significantly.

Comment

The combination of hypertension and hypokalaemia should always prompt consideration of hyperaldosteronism. While hypokalaemia is common in such cases, it is worth remembering that some patients may have normal potassium, even with unilateral adenoma. Early recognition is essential, since surgical treatment of adenoma may correct the biochemical abnormality and improve blood pressure control.

This case also illustrates the importance of not dismissing 'minor' laboratory abnormalities, as they may reveal serious underlying conditions. The patient's persistence in seeking good blood pressure control, coupled with careful investigation and specialist collaboration, ultimately uncovered the root cause.

Lesson Learned

Persistent hypokalaemia in a hypertensive patient without gastrointestinal loss must raise suspicion of hyperaldosteronism. Diuretics are a frequent cause of low potassium in patients treated for high blood pressure, but persistence despite stopping medication suggests another cause. In primary hyperaldosteronism, hypokalaemia is common but not universal, and the diagnosis should not be excluded or approved on the basis of potassium level. This case is a reminder that attention to detail, persistence, and timely referral can lead to a diagnosis that changes the patient's trajectory and offers the possibility of definitive treatment.

Case Study 25

Difficulty in Swallowing

The patient was a 62-year-old Caucasian woman, a retired primary school teacher. At the age of 60 she had stepped down from teaching, having worked for many years with young children, and was now enjoying life in retirement. She never smoked, but occasionally drank wine, usually no more than twice a week. She lived with her husband, also retired, in a private bungalow, and together they shared a contented and settled life. They had one grown-up daughter, herself working as a teacher. The patient was well known to our practice, attending mainly for blood pressure reviews and routine check-ups.

She presented to our practice after booking an appointment, complaining of increasing difficulty in swallowing, a problem she had been noticing for several weeks. She also reported that she had lost approximately one stone in weight over the same period. When asked whether drinking liquids helped to clear food from her throat, she gave an interesting response – fluids did not help very much, which she herself found unusual. She did not complain of nausea, vomiting, haematemesis, or abdominal pain. There was no change in bowel habit, no rectal bleeding, and no urinary symptoms.

Her past medical history included long-standing hypertension, for which she had been taking atenolol 50 mg daily for several years. She had also undergone a hysterectomy for post-menopausal bleeding, which had proved benign. She had no known allergies and no significant family history of major illnesses. Apart from hypertension, she had generally been healthy and had not required hospital care in recent years.

On examination she appeared somewhat frail, with visible weight loss, but she did not look clinically anaemic. She was not short of breath and showed no clinical signs of cyanosis. Her temperature was 37.2°C. Pulse was 88 beats per minute, in sinus rhythm. Blood pressure measured 135/78 mmHg. Cardiovascular and respiratory examinations revealed no abnormality. Abdominal, upper-limb, and lower-limb examinations also showed no clinical signs of pathology. Neurological assessment at that stage was unremarkable, and her cranial nerves appeared intact.

Given her age and her presenting symptom of dysphagia, we considered her case urgent. I immediately contacted a consultant gastroenterologist and was able to secure an urgent appointment. The patient was seen within a week. The consultant's report came back stating that no pathology had been identified at that stage. An oesophagogastroduodenoscopy showed no oesophageal stricture or tumour, and no gastric abnormality. However, her condition did not improve.

She returned to see us again, now complaining of new symptoms. She had developed a hoarse voice and was experiencing increasing difficulty in speaking. These additional features prompted an urgent referral to an ENT surgeon. Within a week she was reviewed, and again no obvious pathology was found in the pharynx, larynx, or tongue. The only observation made was sluggish movement of the vocal cords, and the case was referred back to us.

At this point her story was becoming more concerning. The progression from dysphagia to dysphonia, combined with weight loss, suggested a systemic or neurological disorder rather than a primary ENT or gastrointestinal cause.

Key Questions

1. **What could be the underlying diagnosis in this lady?**
2. **What would be the best management plan?**

Her symptoms, unfortunately, progressed further. Within days she completely lost her voice, while her dysphagia worsened. She came again, asking what she should do. She was advised to go immediately to Accident and Emergency, where she could be assessed further and referred to the appropriate specialty.

At the hospital she was admitted under the medical team. The consultant physician reviewed her case and, after reading her history and the sequence of referrals, requested a second opinion from a neurologist. The neurologist attended the ward promptly. During his examination he immediately noted fasciculations of the tongue, as well as wasting and fasciculation in the small muscles of her right hand. This, together with her dysphagia, dysarthria, and dysphonia, pointed strongly towards a neurological condition.

Final Diagnosis

Motor neurone disease (progressive bulbar palsy).

The findings were discussed with the patient and her husband. Sadly, there was no curative treatment. She was discharged home with arrangements for supportive care, including referral to the multidisciplinary motor neurone disease clinic, where input from physiotherapy, speech therapy, dietetics, and palliative care was coordinated.

Comment

This case was a sobering reminder of how serious neurological disease may present initially with seemingly minor complaints. Dysphagia in an older patient should always be taken seriously, but the lack of gastrointestinal findings could easily have diverted attention. The development of hoarseness and then complete loss of voice provided an important additional clue, directing attention towards neurology rather than ENT or gastroenterology alone.

The delay in diagnosis was not due to lack of vigilance but rather to the insidious and progressive nature of motor neurone disease. Each specialist saw her at a stage where signs were still subtle. It was only when fasciculations and muscle wasting became apparent that the unifying diagnosis was revealed.

Lesson Learned

This was not a common case, yet it remains highly educational. Although motor neurone disease is relatively rare, its initial manifestations can present to a GP, often in non-specific ways. The progressive nature of her symptoms – from dysphagia to dysarthria and finally dysphonia – should serve as a clinical clue. Although rare, such a triad may point towards motor neurone disease, particularly bulbar-onset disease.

The case highlights the importance of persistence and vigilance in the diagnostic process. Even when early specialist assessments find no pathology, the GP must remain alert to the possibility of evolving disease. It also underlines the role of good communication between different specialties, and the importance of ensuring continuity of care, so that evolving symptoms are not overlooked.

Management of such cases goes far beyond medical treatment. Motor neurone disease does not impair memory or intellect, meaning patients remain fully aware of their diagnosis and prognosis. This creates a need for exceptional emotional support, alongside physical supportive measures, both for the patient and their family. For us as GPs, this case represented a profound learning exercise. It reminded us that behind every symptom there may lie a progressive neurological illness, and that support, empathy, and timely referrals can make a significant difference in the patient's journey.

This case demonstrates how symptoms and signs evolve over time. From the first referral to the final diagnosis, the clinical picture changed significantly. Once the situation became clearer, the neurologist was able to reach the diagnosis. This is an important lesson for all clinicians: to remain open to re-evaluating a patient's condition as new features appear, rather than assuming that earlier negative findings exclude a serious underlying disease.

Case Study 26

Recurrent Dizziness

This case was seen in 1980, shortly after I started my post as a medical registrar. The patient was a 46-year-old gentleman who had been working for British Telecom for many years. He was married with two children, aged nine and 11, and lived happily with his family in a semi-detached house in the suburbs. His wife was supportive, and he had a stable home life. He smoked 20 cigarettes daily for the past 15 years but did not drink alcohol. His past medical history included a tonsillectomy at the age of five for recurrent tonsillitis and an appendicectomy at the age of ten. He had no known allergies.

He presented with a history of recurrent dizziness that had persisted for about a year. The episodes occurred without obvious provocation, lasted briefly, and then settled on their own. At first, he regarded them as minor inconveniences and did not seek medical attention. There was no associated ear pain, discharge, or history of ear infections. He had not experienced vomiting or palpitations. Initially, the episodes were infrequent and did not trouble him greatly. Eventually, he consulted his GP, who prescribed medication – likely an antihistamine such as cinnarizine – on the presumption of a vestibular cause. The symptoms persisted intermittently, and six months prior to admission, his GP referred him to an ENT surgeon. No abnormalities were found, and he was discharged back to his GP.

A few days before his hospital admission, the dizziness became more troublesome. He had never collapsed, fainted, or developed chest pain, but the increased frequency of the episodes led him to attend Accident and Emergency, where the case was referred to us as the medical team on call. His family history was negative for any relevant illness, particularly cardiovascular disease or sudden death.

On examination, he appeared well, with no breathlessness, anaemia, or cyanosis. He was comfortable and not in acute distress. His pulse rate was 80 beats per minute and described as irregularly irregular. Blood pressure was 140/78 mmHg. Cardiac examination revealed a very soft ejection systolic murmur in the aortic area, but there were no signs of cardiac failure or clinical cardiomegaly. His respiratory system was unremarkable. Neurological examination showed an alert, comfortable man with no stress-related features. Upper and lower limbs, as well as cranial nerves, were normal. There were no carotid bruits. Abdominal examination revealed no organomegaly or other significant findings.

Routine blood tests were performed. Thyroid function, full blood count, liver function, renal function, calcium, and electrolytes were all within normal limits (urea 6, creatinine 90, sodium 140). An ECG confirmed atrial fibrillation, which was consistent with the irregularly irregular pulse noted on clinical examination.

Key Questions

1. **What do you think the differential diagnosis is?**
2. **How do you manage this case?**
3. **What do you think was the diagnosis?**

At this stage, the combination of atrial fibrillation and recurrent dizziness raised several possibilities. Could the dizziness be due to intermittent cerebral hypoperfusion? Was this a paroxysmal arrhythmia that had stabilised by the time of admission? Could the irregular pulse have been long-standing and unrelated to the dizziness? Other considerations included anaemia, metabolic disturbances, or an undetected structural cardiac problem. The normal blood tests excluded anaemia, thyroid dysfunction, and electrolyte imbalance, narrowing the focus back onto the cardiovascular system.

After discussion with my consultant about the best way forward, I suggested that we present the case at the weekly medical conference held in the hospital, where several consultants would be present. This was a common practice at the time and provided an opportunity for multidisciplinary learning and collaboration. During the conference one of the consultants recommended referral to a cardiologist, noting that the ENT assessment was normal and that cardiology would have the facilities to pursue the diagnosis further.

We acted on that opinion, and my supervising consultant referred the patient to his colleague in the cardiology department at a nearby university hospital, where the necessary facilities were available. After their assessment, the hospital wrote back to us explaining that they had performed an echocardiogram, which established the diagnosis.

Final Diagnosis

Cardiomyopathy.

The diagnosis explained the patient's atrial fibrillation, recurrent dizziness, and soft systolic murmur. At that time, management options were limited, but the importance of close monitoring, anticoagulation to reduce thromboembolic risk, and specialist follow-up were emphasised.

Comment

This case was an important learning experience. For months the patient's dizziness had been treated as an ENT problem, with antihistamines and reassurance. Yet the root cause lay in his heart. The lesson is that atrial fibrillation, even if not fast or symptomatic, should always prompt a search for underlying structural cardiac disease. The echocardiogram provided the key, revealing cardiomyopathy as the underlying cause.

Lesson Learned

A negative family history does not exclude cardiomyopathy; this patient developed the disease without any hereditary predisposition. In a middle-aged, non-heavy drinker presenting with recurrent dizziness, cardiomyopathy or conduction abnormalities must be considered. Dizziness is often attributed to benign vestibular causes, yet in this case it was the cardinal symptom of a significant cardiac condition.

The presence of atrial fibrillation in an otherwise well man should always trigger a careful search for structural heart disease. The arrhythmia may not always be fast or dramatic, but its association with dizziness was an early clue.

Case Study 27

Shortness of Breath in a 12-Year-Old Boy

A 12-year-old boy arrived in England with his parents and his six-year-old sister. The father had come to the United Kingdom to pursue a PhD in chemistry. The family registered at our practice about three months after their arrival, and both children seemed to be settling well, enjoying their new school life.

The father, however, was deeply concerned about his son's health. He reported that the boy had started complaining of shortness of breath about three months before leaving their home country. At first the symptoms were mild, but gradually he began to struggle with normal activities. He could not walk properly, he could not sit comfortably, and he felt unable to breathe well. Importantly, there was no history of cough, wheezing, or high temperature, yet his breathlessness worsened day by day.

While still abroad, the family consulted two paediatricians. Despite thorough assessment, no clear cause could be found. Investigations available at that time were performed and were reported as normal. The child was reassured and sent home, though his symptoms persisted. After arriving in the UK, the father sought further help and took his son to Accident & Emergency on three separate occasions. Each time basic investigations, including blood tests such as full blood count and liver function tests, were performed. On every visit the results were unremarkable, and the boy was discharged home without a diagnosis.

By the time they registered at our practice, the father described himself as completely lost. He felt as though every attempt to obtain help had been met with closed doors. The child himself was otherwise a cheerful boy with no significant past medical history. There was no important family history, no drug allergies, and no regular medications.

On examination, the boy appeared short of breath at rest. He was tachypnoeic, with a respiratory rate of 28 per minute, and his pulse was 110 beats per minute. His blood pressure measured 100/70 mmHg, and his temperature was 37.6°C. He was not cyanosed and there was no clinical evidence of anaemia. Heart sounds were rapid but without clear murmurs. The jugular venous pressure appeared raised.

Chest examination revealed symmetrical but limited expansion, with central trachea and vesicular breath sounds. There were no added sounds. The abdomen was normal, with no hepatosplenomegaly and no ascites. Neurological examination of the limbs showed normal tone, power, and reflexes. His weight was 14 kilograms and his height 120 centimetres, both low for his age, suggesting poor growth or failure to thrive.

Routine blood tests were arranged. The full blood count was normal, but the ESR was raised at 50 mm/hour. Renal function and liver function were within normal limits, and no obvious abnormality was identified.

Key Questions

1. **What could be the possible differential diagnoses for this child's presentation?**
2. **What should be the immediate action plan for further assessment and management?**
3. **What do you think was the final diagnosis?**

The child and his father were understandably frustrated. His progressive breathlessness was interrupting school, and the family, living in a foreign country, were distressed by his deterioration. Clinically, the picture was confusing. The heart sounds were rather muffled, though without definite murmurs, and nothing conclusive could be found in the community setting.

However, the raised jugular venous pressure was a significant sign. At this point, differential diagnoses included a mediastinal tumour, pericardial effusion, rheumatic fever, pyogenic infection, coxsackievirus infection, tuberculosis, or even a connective tissue disorder such as rheumatoid arthritis or systemic lupus erythematosus.

A mediastinal tumour such as lymphoma could present with progressive dyspnoea by compressing the great veins or airways. Clues might include distended neck veins, facial swelling, or mediastinal widening on chest imaging. A pericardial effusion was strongly suggested by the muffled heart sounds, raised jugular venous pressure, tachycardia, and the absence of focal lung signs, with the elevated ESR supporting an inflammatory cause.

Rheumatic fever was another possibility, given the boy's overseas background, as valvular involvement could result in heart failure. However, the lack of obvious murmurs and no clear history of preceding pharyngitis made this less likely, though early or 'silent' rheumatic carditis could not be entirely excluded.

Infective causes such as bacterial pericarditis needed to be considered, though high fever and systemic illness were not prominent. Viral myocarditis or pericarditis, particularly from coxsackievirus, was another plausible explanation, especially if subtle prodromal symptoms had been overlooked.

Tuberculosis, given the epidemiological risk, remained a leading candidate; tuberculous pericarditis often presents with breathlessness and raised JVP, without cough or wheeze. Finally, systemic conditions such as lupus or juvenile rheumatoid arthritis can present with serositis, including pericardial involvement, and must be considered when no straightforward cause is found.

The case was clearly beyond primary care. I contacted a consultant paediatric cardiologist at a larger centre, explained the situation, and arranged an urgent appointment. The family were greatly relieved to finally have a specialist review.

A week later, I received a detailed letter from the consultant. A series of investigations were undertaken, including chest X-ray, ultrasound, Mantoux test, autoimmune screen, and repeat blood tests. The ESR remained elevated, but other blood results were largely normal. Crucially, echocardiography demonstrated a pericardial effusion. Pericardiocentesis was performed, and blood-stained fluid was aspirated and sent for culture and sensitivity. The Mantoux test was positive, and culture of the aspirated fluid later confirmed the presence of Mycobacterium tuberculosis.

Final Diagnosis

Cardiac tamponade caused by tuberculous pericardial effusion.

Lesson Learned

This case illustrates the importance of persistence when faced with unexplained symptoms, particularly in children who repeatedly attend emergency departments without resolution. Such a pattern should always raise concern for a significant underlying disease. It also underlines the boundaries of general practice and the necessity of recognising when specialist referral is essential. The decision to seek urgent paediatric cardiology input proved to be decisive in this case. Another key lesson is the recognition of growth failure as an important red flag in children.

A 12-year-old boy weighing only 14 kilograms and measuring 120 centimetres should immediately alert the clinician to chronic or systemic disease, even before more specific signs are evident. Finally, the case highlights the need to consider the patient's background. Children arriving from regions such as South Asia, Africa, or the Middle East may present with tuberculosis, which, while relatively uncommon in the United Kingdom, remains endemic in those parts of the world and must remain in the clinician's mind when forming a differential diagnosis.

Case Study 28

Recurrent Abdominal Pain

This case was the wife of one of our patients, who had originally emigrated from South Yemen. He later brought his wife to the United Kingdom for medical attention. She was a 64-year-old lady who did not speak English. She had never smoked, never consumed alcohol, and had lived all her life in Aden, South Yemen. She had four grown-up children and described a happy family life, supported by her husband who regularly sent money home while working abroad.

The onset of her illness was approximately six months before she travelled to the UK. At that time, she began to suffer from recurrent abdominal pain, typically central in location, not radiating to the back, and occurring in an intermittent pattern. Alongside this, she noticed episodes of facial flushing and persistent watery diarrhoea. These symptoms gradually worsened, and she experienced marked weight loss, likely a consequence of chronic diarrhoea. She became increasingly depressed and frustrated, describing her life as dominated by frequent trips to the toilet, abdominal pain, and loss of energy, which rendered her unable to function normally.

During her time in Aden, she had consulted three or four different doctors. She was given symptomatic treatment but no firm diagnosis was reached. Basic investigations, including routine blood tests, X-rays, and abdominal ultrasound, were reportedly performed, but all were unhelpful. She brought these results with her to the UK, but they added little value. Previous medical history was not relevant. She denied any allergy, and she was not taking any regular medication apart from a few painkillers brought from Aden.

On arrival, she joined our practice. On initial examination, she was not clinically anaemic, showed no obvious jaundice, and had no evidence of shortness of breath. However, she was clearly demonstrating signs of weight loss. She measured 162 centimetres in height and weighed 54 kilograms. Her temperature was normal, pulse 100 beats per minute, and blood pressure 110/70 mmHg.

Abdominal examination revealed no palpable masses but there was some tenderness in the right iliac fossa. Bowel sounds were present and not obstructed. Her skin appeared very rough and dry, almost eczematous in character, suggestive of dermatitis. Examination of the limbs was unremarkable. Neurological examination, though limited, was grossly normal.

Initial investigations were performed in our practice. Her haemoglobin was 10 g/dL, consistent with a microcytic, hypochromic anaemia. Platelet count was normal. Liver function tests were abnormal, with raised transaminases, an elevated bilirubin, and a slightly increased alkaline phosphatase. Renal function was entirely normal, with urea and creatinine within range.

At this stage, I felt the case was beyond my scope in primary care. The combination of diarrhoea, weight loss, anaemia, flushing, abnormal liver tests, and skin changes suggested a complex systemic disease. I therefore referred her urgently to a nearby university teaching hospital for further evaluation.

Key Questions

1. **What is the most likely diagnosis and what are the differential diagnoses?**
2. **How should this case be managed?**

From a general practice perspective, the differential diagnosis was wide. One possibility was coeliac disease, as this can present with chronic diarrhoea, malabsorption, weight loss, and anaemia. However, it would not account for flushing and abnormal liver function in this form. Colonic carcinoma was another important consideration, particularly with her age, anaemia, and weight loss. Although carcinoma of the colon may cause diarrhoea and constitutional symptoms, it would not typically explain the flushing episodes.

A small bowel lymphoma was also a possibility. Such tumours may present with diarrhoea, malabsorption, anaemia, and weight loss, and can mimic other gastrointestinal conditions. Infective causes, such as giardiasis, were considered but would not account for flushing or abnormal liver function tests. Inflammatory bowel disease such as Crohn's disease could also present with diarrhoea, abdominal pain, and anaemia, but again the flushing was atypical.

The combination of diarrhoea, weight loss, abnormal liver function, anaemia, skin changes, and – most strikingly – facial flushing suggested a systemic cause. This constellation raised the strong possibility of a neuroendocrine tumour with carcinoid syndrome. In such cases, serotonin and other vasoactive amines are secreted by the tumour, leading to diarrhoea, vasomotor flushing, bronchospasm, and, in some cases, right-sided heart disease. The abnormal liver tests may represent hepatic metastases, as carcinoid hormones are usually metabolised in the liver, and symptoms often emerge only after hepatic spread.

Given the complexity, hospital admission was the appropriate step. She was admitted to a university teaching hospital and underwent extensive investigations over a two-month period. These included CT and MRI scans, PET scanning, and tissue biopsies. Her urine showed markedly elevated 5-HIAA levels, the metabolic breakdown product of serotonin, which strongly supports the diagnosis of carcinoid syndrome. Taken together, the findings confirmed the presence of a neuroendocrine tumour with systemic manifestations.

Final Diagnosis

Carcinoid syndrome due to neuroendocrine tumour, confirmed by elevated 5-HIAA levels.

Lesson Learned

This case emphasises how certain combinations of symptoms can point towards less common but important diagnoses. Chronic diarrhoea and weight loss are frequently encountered in primary care and are often initially attributed to irritable bowel syndrome, coeliac disease, or chronic infection. However, when accompanied by flushing and dermatitis-like skin changes, the diagnostic focus must widen. These additional features, especially when present alongside abnormal liver function tests, strongly suggest a systemic process such as carcinoid syndrome.

It also underlines the need to always consider malignancy in patients with persistent diarrhoea, unexplained weight loss, and anaemia, especially when initial investigations fail to yield an explanation. Although small bowel lymphoma and colonic carcinoma were important differentials, neither would explain the characteristic flushing episodes. That single feature became the crucial clinical clue that directed thinking towards a neuroendocrine process.

Another important lesson is the limitation of primary care investigations in complex systemic illness. While basic blood tests and scans can exclude common conditions, they are often inadequate in detecting neuroendocrine tumours. In such circumstances, timely referral to secondary or tertiary care is essential. This patient required specialist imaging, tissue sampling, and biochemical testing of 5-HIAA, which could not have been provided in the community.

From a psychosocial angle, this case also highlights the added challenge of language barriers. The patient relied on her husband for interpretation, and while this was helpful, subtle details may have been lost. Professional medical interpretation could have provided greater clarity in describing her symptoms. Furthermore, her frustration and depression were aggravated both by her illness and by the difficulties of navigating healthcare in a foreign system.

Finally, this case demonstrates the importance of recognising red-flag symptoms – particularly unexplained weight loss, persistent diarrhoea, and systemic features such as flushing. These must never be underestimated. They demand urgent and thorough investigation. Early recognition and appropriate referral can greatly improve diagnostic accuracy and patient outcomes.

Case Study 29

Jaundice and Shortness of Breath

This case was seen in 1979 in North Wales, while I was working in medicine in that region. The patient was a 62-year-old retired farmer who had stopped working two years earlier. He lived with his wife, who herself had retired from her clerical post in the local hospital. Together they enjoyed a quiet and settled lifestyle. Their weekly routine was simple but fulfilling: they attended church every Sunday, went to the pub twice a week, and socialised regularly with neighbours and members of the local farming community. Although they never drank to excess, these social occasions gave them joy and connection. They had three grown-up children, two of whom still lived nearby and visited once or twice a week. The couple were content, sociable, and well supported by family and friends.

The man's presentation began when his family noticed he appeared unusually yellow. At around the same time, he himself began to feel increasingly short of breath. Concerned, his general practitioner arranged for his direct admission to hospital. The patient, though aware of his breathlessness, had not recognised any other specific problems. He denied dark urine, pale stools, abdominal pain, rectal bleeding, or haematemesis. He did, however, report increasing tiredness and a sense of generalised exhaustion that interfered with his daily activities.

His past medical history was notable. He had long-standing hypertension, managed with methyldopa and atenolol 50 mg daily. Three years earlier he had undergone a hip replacement, from which he had recovered well. More significantly, five years earlier he had been diagnosed with carcinoma of the bowel, which had been treated with surgical resection followed by chemotherapy. He was considered to be in remission. He also suffered from psoriasis with associated psoriatic arthritis, using ibuprofen and co-proxamol for pain control. His allergy history included rubber and penicillin, both longstanding.

On examination he was a pleasant, cooperative man, 176 centimetres in height and weighing 70 kilograms. He was visibly jaundiced, though not breathless at rest. His temperature was normal. His pulse was 90 beats per minute in sinus rhythm, and his blood pressure measured 145/90 mmHg. Cardiovascular examination revealed normal heart sounds with no murmurs, extra sounds, or signs of failure. Respiratory examination was unremarkable: chest expansion was good, breath sounds were vesicular, and there were no added sounds. He had no palpable lymphadenopathy in the neck or groin.

Abdominal examination revealed no tenderness. The liver and spleen were not palpable, there was no organomegaly, and no abdominal masses were detected. His skin showed the classic psoriatic plaques over the elbows and knees, with joint deformities consistent with psoriatic arthritis affecting both knees. Neurological examination was grossly normal: he was alert, oriented, and motor and sensory systems were intact.

At this stage, the presence of jaundice with relatively few other clinical findings necessitated a broad differential diagnosis and a wide range of investigations. A chest X-ray was arranged to exclude pulmonary or mediastinal pathology. Blood tests included full liver function, viral serology for hepatitis B and C, and a peripheral blood film. An abdominal X-ray was also requested to evaluate for gallstones.

The results became available within a few days. The chest and abdominal X-rays were both normal. Blood results revealed a haemoglobin level of 10 g/dL, indicating anaemia. Importantly, the reticulocyte count was markedly raised at 15 per cent. Bilirubin was elevated, yet liver enzymes remained within normal limits.

Key Questions

1. **What is the differential diagnosis in this case?**
2. **How should it be managed?**
3. **What is the final diagnosis?**

The differential diagnosis for an older man presenting with jaundice, anaemia, and a raised reticulocyte count was carefully considered. Haemolytic anaemia was immediately high on the list. This could arise through autoimmune mechanisms, drug reactions, or secondary to systemic conditions such as connective tissue disease. Drug-induced haemolysis, in particular, needed to be considered, given his medication history.

Viral hepatitis was another important possibility, particularly as jaundice and anaemia can coexist in viral infection. For this reason, hepatitis serology had been arranged. Obstructive causes such as gallstones, cholangiocarcinoma, or other hepatic malignancy also had to be excluded. In an older patient, the possibility of recurrent disease from his previous bowel carcinoma could not be ignored, as metastatic infiltration of the liver may present with jaundice and anaemia.

However, the results of the investigations narrowed the possibilities significantly. The raised bilirubin, together with a markedly elevated reticulocyte count, pointed strongly towards a haemolytic process rather than hepatic or obstructive disease. The fact that liver enzymes remained normal supported this interpretation. The normal abdominal imaging effectively excluded gallstones or gross hepatic infiltration. Taken together, these findings indicated that the jaundice was pre-hepatic in origin – the result of increased haemolysis rather than impaired liver function or bile duct obstruction.

Given his medication history, methyldopa emerged as the most likely trigger. At that time, methyldopa was widely prescribed as an antihypertensive but was already well known to cause immune-mediated haemolytic anaemia. The raised reticulocyte count confirmed the bone marrow's attempt to compensate for red cell destruction. A direct Coombs test, had it been performed, would almost certainly have confirmed the autoimmune mechanism.

Final Diagnosis

Haemolytic anaemia caused by methyldopa.

Lesson Learned

This case highlights the importance of a structured and logical approach to jaundice. In older adults, it is easy to assume a hepatic or obstructive cause such as gallstones, viral hepatitis, or malignancy. However, the presence of anaemia together with a raised reticulocyte count should immediately direct the clinician's mind towards haemolysis. Careful interpretation of basic blood results provided the crucial clue in this case.

The case also underlines the value of reviewing the drug history meticulously. Methyldopa, although effective for hypertension, is a well-recognised cause of immune haemolytic anaemia. Identifying this link not only prevents unnecessary and invasive investigations but also ensures timely and effective management.

The central management step is immediate withdrawal of the offending drug. Supportive measures such as transfusion may be required, and referral to haematology is appropriate for further monitoring and advice. Replacement antihypertensive therapy should be instituted to maintain blood pressure control.

Another important reflection is how past medical history can initially distract the clinician. In this patient, previous bowel carcinoma could easily have led one to suspect recurrence or hepatic metastasis as the cause of jaundice. Without careful consideration of the blood results, the diagnosis might have been delayed or missed. Similarly, gallstones are common in this age group, and without the reticulocyte finding, an obstructive cause may have been incorrectly pursued.

Finally, this case demonstrates the need for clinicians to remain alert to pre-hepatic causes of jaundice. While the mind often jumps to liver disease or biliary obstruction, haemolysis is an equally important cause, particularly in the presence of anaemia and a raised reticulocyte count. Recognising this distinction allows for accurate diagnosis and avoids both misdirection and unnecessary procedures.

Case Study 30

Double Vision

I was not directly involved in this case, but I found it interesting enough to include. The patient was a 25-year-old man whom I met briefly while on holiday in the Middle East. Through relatives I was visiting he approached me, hoping that as a doctor from the United Kingdom I might help. He had been struggling for around eight months without a clear diagnosis.

He was a married man with a five-year-old child. He worked as an accountant, did not smoke, did not drink alcohol, and lived a quiet family life. Despite his youth and health, his unexplained condition was beginning to dominate his day-to-day activities and cause significant distress.

His story went back seven to eight months. He began to suffer from episodes of double vision, which appeared suddenly and without warning. The diplopia was not associated with headache, seizures, or pain. Curiously, the symptom would disappear after a night's sleep. In the mornings he was normal, but as the day progressed the double vision returned, particularly when he was tired.

He consulted an ophthalmologist who carried out a thorough examination but found no abnormality. When symptoms persisted, a senior ophthalmologist also reviewed him and again found no pathology. He was reassured and sent home, the problem briefly settled, but soon returned.

Frustrated, he sought further advice and was referred to a physician. The physician examined him comprehensively: his blood pressure, pulse, cardiovascular system, and neurological system were all found to be normal. Routine blood investigations, including full blood count, kidney function, and liver function tests, were also normal. Again, he was told there was no clear abnormality. The young man went home dissatisfied, feeling his symptoms were being dismissed as anxiety or stress.

His past medical history gave some important background. He had been diagnosed with hypothyroidism three years earlier and was taking thyroxine 100 micrograms daily. He had also experienced alopecia areata on his scalp, which had later regrown, and white depigmented patches on his hands extending to his arms, consistent with vitiligo. These conditions suggested an autoimmune tendency, though at the time nobody had linked them with his current symptoms. He was not allergic to any medications.

When I met him through my relatives, I had no equipment and could not perform an examination. I listened carefully to his account instead. What struck me was the precise pattern of his symptoms. The double vision appeared in the afternoons, worsened when he was tired or recovering from an infection such as influenza, and resolved after rest. At times, he also experienced weakness, struggling to comb his hair or to speak clearly. He told me, 'Doctor, I don't understand why I feel weak, have double vision, and can't speak properly.'

The story was unusual and important. Though neurology was not my area of specialty, the history strongly suggested a neuromuscular disorder. The fluctuating weakness, the diurnal variation, and the ocular and bulbar involvement pointed in one direction. I discussed the case with a local physician I knew, explained the history, and stressed that this young man required further specialist testing.

Key Questions

1. **What is the differential diagnosis in this case?**
2. **How should this patient be investigated and managed?**
3. **What is the final diagnosis?**

The differential diagnosis of fluctuating weakness and intermittent diplopia in a young adult is wide. Multiple sclerosis (MS) was a consideration, as it can produce diplopia and weakness, but in MS the deficits tend to persist and accumulate rather than fluctuate with fatigue. Furthermore, additional neurological signs would typically be present.

Thyroid eye disease was another possibility, particularly as he had hypothyroidism. However, thyroid eye disease usually produces proptosis, lid retraction, or obvious ophthalmopathy, none of which were seen.

Primary myopathies, such as polymyositis or mitochondrial disorders, can cause weakness, but they tend not to show such dramatic fluctuation or isolated ocular and bulbar involvement.

Functional neurological disorders also had to be considered, especially given normal initial examinations, but the consistency of the symptom pattern and the clear association with fatigue made a functional cause much less likely.

The features most in keeping with his condition were those of myasthenia gravis. The fluctuating diplopia, worsening with exertion, improving after rest, and the associated bulbar weakness (difficulty speaking, combing hair) were highly suggestive. His autoimmune background - hypothyroidism, alopecia, and vitiligo - further reinforced the possibility.

He was referred to a specialised hospital where he underwent a comprehensive series of investigations. These included antibody studies, which demonstrated acetylcholine receptor antibodies, and imaging of the mediastinum, which revealed a thymoma. He was also started on anticholinesterase medication under careful supervision, with intravenous atropine 0.5-1 mg kept available as a safeguard. The response to therapy supported the clinical suspicion. Taken together, the investigations confirmed the diagnosis.

Final Diagnosis

Myasthenia gravis associated with thymoma.

Lesson Learned

This case demonstrates the crucial importance of listening attentively to the patient's history. Despite multiple normal examinations and negative routine tests, the diagnosis lay in the pattern of symptoms he described. The fluctuating weakness, the ocular and bulbar involvement, and the improvement with rest are classic for myasthenia gravis.

It also shows the significance of linking past medical history to new symptoms. His hypothyroidism, alopecia, and vitiligo all indicated an autoimmune diathesis. Recognising that myasthenia gravis is often associated with other autoimmune conditions can help guide the clinician, even when examination offers no clues.

The case further underlines the role of specialist centres in confirming such diagnoses. Myasthenia gravis requires antibody testing, electrophysiological studies, and often mediastinal imaging to detect thymoma. These investigations are beyond the scope of primary care and demonstrate the importance of referral when suspicion is high.

Management also provides key lessons. Anticholinesterase medications must be started in hospital, with atropine available to counteract adverse cholinergic reactions. In patients with thymoma, surgical removal is often indicated. Long-term management may involve immunosuppression and careful monitoring.

Above all, this case highlights that careful history-taking remains the cornerstone of diagnosis. Even when initial tests and examinations are unrevealing, the patient's narrative may contain the essential diagnostic clues. For this young man, being listened to and taken seriously provided both relief and a path to definitive treatment.

Case Study 31

Recurrent Mouth Ulcers

This case concerned a 37-year-old Kurdish man who had immigrated from Iraq ten years earlier. He was married with two children, aged seven and nine, and lived with his family in a council house. He never smoked, did not drink alcohol, and overall lived a stable family life with his wife, although he was unemployed at the time.

His main complaint was recurrent painful mouth ulcers, which had troubled him for about 18 months. These ulcers were typical aphthous lesions, lasting for several days before healing, only to recur repeatedly. He had attended his GP on several occasions and was prescribed topical steroids, which provided temporary relief but no lasting cure. The ulcers became an accepted part of his life, though they continued to cause pain and frustration.

After registering with our practice, his symptoms expanded. He developed eye pain and blurred vision, which led him to the local eye hospital. There he was diagnosed with uveitis and treated with steroid eye drops, after which his vision gradually improved. While under our care, he also developed a painful red rash on both shins, clinically consistent with erythema nodosum. A chest X-ray was performed to exclude tuberculosis and sarcoidosis, but no abnormality was found.

Soon afterwards, the patient experienced recurrent genital ulcers, which lasted for several weeks before resolving. In addition, he began to develop joint pains, particularly in the knees and hands. At that time there was no definite evidence of reactive arthritis, but the musculoskeletal involvement was undeniable.

Blood tests - including full blood count, renal and liver function - were all within normal limits. However, inflammatory markers were raised, with an ESR of 40 mm/hr and CRP of 35 mg/L. He had no systemic upset such as fever or night sweats, but the oral ulcers remained frequent and painful.

Over the following four to five weeks the patient developed abdominal pain. It was persistent, resistant to simple analgesia, not radiating, and not associated with vomiting. Its cause remained unclear despite repeated assessments.

His past medical history was otherwise unremarkable. He had no drug allergies and was not on regular medication apart from occasional topical steroids and the steroid eye drops prescribed for his uveitis.

On clinical examination, he appeared well and was cooperative, though communication was occasionally difficult because he spoke limited English. He was 178 centimetres tall and weighed 79 kilograms. There was no evidence of anaemia or cyanosis, and his temperature was normal. Blood pressure measured 140/80 mmHg and his pulse was 89 beats per minute in sinus rhythm. Cardiovascular and respiratory examinations were unremarkable. The abdomen was soft with no palpable hepatosplenomegaly or lymphadenopathy. His legs showed residual pigmentation from previous erythema nodosum. Peripheral pulses and reflexes were intact, and neurological examination revealed no abnormality.

Subsequent investigations confirmed persistently raised inflammatory markers, with ESR of 54 mm/hr and CRP of 40 mg/L. His haemoglobin level was 10.5 g/dL, showing a normocytic, normochromic anaemia. Kidney and liver function remained normal, and urinalysis showed no proteinuria or haematuria.

Key Questions

1. **What is the differential diagnosis in this case?**
2. **How should this patient be investigated and managed?**
3. **What is the final diagnosis?**

The differential diagnosis was initially wide. Recurrent oral ulcers could simply represent chronic aphthous stomatitis, but the persistence and severity raised suspicion of an underlying systemic disorder. Haematological causes such as iron deficiency or leukopenia were considered but excluded through testing.

The uveitis suggested an inflammatory or autoimmune condition. Reactive arthritis (formerly Reiter's syndrome) was a possibility, especially when considered alongside arthritis and mucocutaneous involvement. However, genital ulcers are not typical of reactive arthritis.

The erythema nodosum broadened the possibilities further, raising consideration of sarcoidosis, inflammatory bowel disease, or other systemic inflammatory conditions. Abdominal pain introduced the possibility of Crohn's disease, yet he did not report diarrhoea, gastrointestinal bleeding, or significant weight loss.

When viewed together, the constellation of symptoms - recurrent mouth and genital ulcers, uveitis, erythema nodosum, arthritis, and abdominal pain - pointed strongly to a single multisystem disorder. The unifying diagnosis was Behçet's disease, a chronic relapsing inflammatory condition characterised by recurrent oral and genital ulcers, ocular involvement, skin lesions, and variable systemic manifestations including arthritis and gastrointestinal disease.

The case was clearly beyond the scope of general practice. He was referred to rheumatology, which coordinated his care alongside dermatology and ophthalmology. Further investigations continued to show raised ESR and CRP and a hypochromic normocytic anaemia. Renal and hepatic function remained intact. A biopsy of an oral ulcer showed only non-specific inflammation but was not diagnostic. Despite this, the overall clinical picture was highly characteristic.

After multidisciplinary review, the diagnosis of Behçet's disease was made. Treatment began with topical measures for the ulcers, but these were inadequate. The patient was started on systemic corticosteroids, followed later by long-term immunosuppressive therapy with azathioprine. As the disease progressed, he required escalation to cyclophosphamide. Because of the risks associated with cyclophosphamide, he needed weekly monitoring of blood counts and liver function, coordinated between hospital and primary care.

Final Diagnosis

Behçet's disease.

Lesson Learned

This case illustrates how apparently unrelated symptoms across different systems may, when carefully considered, reveal a unifying diagnosis. Recurrent mouth ulcers may at first appear trivial, but when associated with uveitis, genital ulcers, erythema nodosum, arthritis, and abdominal pain, they point clearly towards Behçet's disease.

The case also underlines the importance of recognising multisystem patterns. Treating each symptom in isolation - oral ulcers by the dentist, uveitis by the ophthalmologist, arthritis by the GP - would fragment the picture. It was only by linking these features together that the true systemic nature of the illness became apparent.

Another lesson is the necessity of multidisciplinary collaboration. Effective management of Behçet's disease requires coordination between rheumatology, ophthalmology, dermatology, and general practice. Long-term immunosuppressive therapy carries risks, making close monitoring of blood and liver function essential.

The case also reminds us that patients with limited English proficiency face extra barriers in communicating their symptoms. Careful listening, patience, and sometimes the use of interpreters are crucial to avoid missing important details.

Finally, the case demonstrates how inflammatory conditions can evolve over time. Behçet's disease may first appear as recurrent oral ulcers, but later reveal its multisystem nature. Persistence in following up patients and recognising new patterns ensures early referral and appropriate treatment, preventing serious complications such as vision loss or gastrointestinal perforation.

Case Study 32

Dorsum of Hand Recurrent Skin Eruption

This case concerned a 25-year-old dentist who had recently qualified and was working in London. He remained registered with our practice as his GP. He was young, active, and dynamic, with no history of smoking or alcohol use. At weekends he returned home to stay with his parents, travelling back to London for work during the week. Apart from the occasional coughs and colds, he had always enjoyed good health and had no significant medical history.

The story began shortly after his return from a holiday in Barcelona with friends. He had spent time swimming in the Mediterranean and lying on the beach. On returning to the UK, he attended my surgery to show me a skin eruption over the dorsum of his right hand. The rash had appeared suddenly, was intensely itchy, and resembled contact dermatitis. At first glance, I could not be certain of the cause. Because of the recent beach exposure, I considered whether this might have been a jellyfish sting. I prescribed a topical steroid cream (1 per cent hydrocortisone) together with an antihistamine. For reassurance, I contacted a dermatologist and sent him a photograph. The dermatologist supported the impression of a possible jellyfish reaction.

The lesion settled with treatment. However, a day or two later, an identical eruption reappeared in precisely the same location. The patient returned over the weekend, perplexed. I reviewed the history again, including any exposures in his dental practice, but nothing obvious was identified. The rash once again improved with antihistamines and topical steroid.

Soon, a curious pattern emerged. When he stayed at home with his parents over the weekend, the skin cleared completely. Yet each time he returned to London for work on Monday, the lesion reappeared. This cycle repeated itself for several weeks. His past medical history remained unremarkable. He was not taking any regular medication other than the antihistamine and reported no known allergies.

On examination, he was well in himself. The only abnormal finding was the rash over the dorsum of his right hand. The rest of his skin was entirely clear, with no lesions elsewhere on the body. Systemic examination, including cardiovascular, respiratory, and abdominal systems, was completely normal.

Key Questions

1. **What do you think might be the problem?**
2. **What is the appropriate action plan?**
3. **What is the final diagnosis?**

Because of the clear temporal relationship with his working week, the pattern strongly suggested an occupational trigger. I spoke to him again and asked specifically about the materials he was handling in the dental surgery. He explained that he always wore gloves and therefore did not think his hands had been exposed to bonding agents or gels.

Later, he sent me a list of the materials he had been using at work. Among them was Optibond, a dental bonding gel. Reviewing its components, I discovered that it contained methacrylate compounds, which are well-recognised skin sensitisers. Importantly, methacrylates are able to penetrate latex gloves, the type he had been using routinely. By contrast, nitrile gloves provide an effective barrier against these chemicals.

This insight proved decisive. He switched from latex to nitrile gloves and carefully avoided further contact with the bonding gel. The rash resolved completely and did not recur. This simple but targeted intervention confirmed the diagnosis.

The initial differential diagnosis was wide. Given the recent Mediterranean holiday, my first thought was an acute jellyfish sting or some other marine reaction. The rash was itchy, localised, and sudden, which made this plausible. A second possibility was photodermatitis, a reaction to sunlight exposure, sometimes intensified by medications or contact with plant products. Another consideration was insect bites, which may present with localised itchy rashes.

However, the repeating cycle provided the most important clue. The rash disappeared completely when he was away from work and reappeared only during the working week in London. This pointed firmly to an occupational cause, particularly contact dermatitis. The discovery of methacrylate in Optibond, combined with the knowledge that these chemicals penetrate latex gloves, refined the diagnosis to occupational allergic contact dermatitis caused by methacrylate exposure.

Final Diagnosis

Occupational contact dermatitis due to methacrylate exposure, penetrating latex gloves.

Lesson Learned

This case illustrates several important clinical lessons.

Firstly, it emphasises the importance of careful, detailed history-taking, particularly regarding occupational exposures. The recurring cycle of resolution at weekends and recurrence during the working week was the decisive clue. Had this pattern not been noticed, the diagnosis might have remained elusive.

Secondly, it demonstrates the value of considering occupational dermatology. In young professionals such as dentists, early recognition of work-related skin conditions is crucial. Without intervention, persistent exposure can result in chronic dermatitis and, in some cases, force patients to abandon their chosen careers.

Thirdly, the case highlights the need to understand the limitations of protective equipment. Latex gloves are widely assumed to provide universal protection, but in fact certain chemicals, including methacrylates, can pass through them. Nitrile gloves, by contrast, provide the necessary protection. For dentists, dental nurses, and others regularly handling bonding agents or acrylic resins, this knowledge is essential.

Finally, the case illustrates the process of refining a differential diagnosis. Initially, the holiday history led me to consider jellyfish stings, photodermatitis, or insect bites. Only by reviewing the temporal pattern and occupational history did the true cause emerge. This demonstrates the principle that a broad differential diagnosis should be entertained at first, but must then be narrowed by carefully correlating the clinical story with exposures and circumstances.

In the end, what began as a trivial looking skin rash carried significant implications. By recognising the occupational cause early, we were able to prevent a young dentist's temporary irritation from becoming a lifelong disability.

Case Study 33

Raised Serum Creatine Kinase

A 42-year-old man worked as a locum radiologist for the NHS, moving between hospitals on fixed-term contracts. Although he had been on our practice list for several years, his work frequently took him away from the area, and when he was working elsewhere he often registered temporarily with local GPs. He was married to a medical secretary employed at the same hospital where I practised, and they had two children, aged seven and nine, both attending private school. He had never smoked and only occasionally drank alcohol at social events.

The reason for his consultation was an abnormal blood result obtained outside our practice: a raised creatine kinase (CK). A few months earlier he had opted for a private general health check that included routine tests such as weight, blood pressure, lipid profile, renal and liver function, and HbA1c. At that time he was informed that his HbA1c was 45 mmol/mol, placing him in the pre-diabetic range. Motivated by this finding, he decided to improve his lifestyle and began attending the gym daily for vigorous exercise.

Several months later, while working in the north of England, repeat blood tests revealed a CK level of 950 IU/L. Disturbed by the result, he contacted our practice and arranged an appointment for review.

On consultation, he denied myalgia, cramps, weakness, or tenderness. There had been no trauma, no recent intramuscular injections, no viral illnesses, and he was not taking statins or any other myotoxic drugs. He reported feeling well, enjoying his work, and maintaining his new exercise routine.

Examination was unremarkable. His height was 178 centimetres and his weight 80 kilograms. His pulse was regular at 80 beats per minute, and his blood pressure was 145/70 mmHg. Cardiovascular examination revealed normal heart sounds with no murmurs. Respiratory examination showed clear breath sounds and good expansion. His abdomen was soft, non-tender, with no organomegaly. A neurological screen was entirely normal, with no evidence of weakness or sensory loss. Urinalysis was negative for blood and protein.

I arranged confirmatory investigations. Liver enzymes and alkaline phosphatase were normal. Full blood count showed a haemoglobin of 13.8 g/dL with normal indices. His lipid profile was favourable, with a total cholesterol of 4 mmol/L and normal triglycerides. Renal function was normal. Repeat CK measured 957 IU/L, confirming the earlier abnormal result.

Key Questions

1. **What is the differential diagnosis in this case?**
2. **How should this case be managed?**
3. **What is the final diagnosis?**

The history and results prompted a structured consideration of raised creatine kinase.

Neurological causes: central nervous system injury, seizures, or neuromuscular disorders can elevate CK, but these are usually associated with neurological deficits. None were present here.

Other systemic causes: malignant hyperthermia, endocrine disorders (such as Cushing's or Addison's), and certain infections can all produce CK elevation, though they usually present with additional symptoms.

Given the absence of muscle pain, tenderness, weakness, or neurological abnormalities, and with normal renal and hepatic function, most serious pathologies were unlikely. The only relevant change in his lifestyle was the initiation of a daily, high-intensity exercise regimen.

Management

In primary care, the management of an asymptomatic adult with raised CK follows a structured approach. The first priority is to confirm the abnormality, exclude laboratory error, and check renal function to rule out rhabdomyolysis risk. This had already been achieved: CK was consistently elevated at ~950 IU/L, but renal function and urinalysis were normal.

The next step is to identify potential reversible causes such as exercise, medications, or recent trauma. In this case, the temporal link between the rise in CK and the start of vigorous daily workouts was compelling. Exercise-induced hyperCKaemia is well recognised, especially in individuals who are unaccustomed to sustained high-intensity activity.

Guidelines recommend rest from strenuous exercise for 5-7 days, adequate hydration, and repeat testing. If CK levels normalise or fall significantly, the elevation can be attributed to benign, exercise-related muscle breakdown. If levels remain persistently raised (especially >1,500-2,000 IU/L) or if symptoms develop, further investigations are warranted. These would include thyroid function tests, autoimmune screens, viral serology, and referral to neurology or rheumatology for more advanced assessment.

For this patient, reassurance was key. We advised him to stop strenuous exercise temporarily, maintain hydration, and repeat CK after a week of rest. We discussed the importance of sustainable, graded exercise rather than daily high-intensity workouts, particularly as his motivation had been to control pre-diabetes. A balanced programme of aerobic activity, strength training, and rest days would be both safer and more effective long-term.

Final Diagnosis

Exercise-induced elevation of creatine kinase (benign hyperCKaemia).

Lesson Learned

This case demonstrates that not all abnormal blood results indicate serious disease. A raised CK can cause considerable anxiety, particularly for health professionals such as this radiologist, who are acutely aware of the potential implications. However, it is important to interpret laboratory results in context.

A structured approach to CK elevation is essential: confirm the abnormality, review the drug and exercise history, assess for muscle or cardiac symptoms, and check renal function. Only if results remain persistently abnormal or symptoms emerge should more invasive investigations be pursued.

This case also highlights the role of lifestyle change in medicine. Motivated by a borderline HbA1c, the patient embraced exercise enthusiastically. While this was commendable, unaccustomed and intense workouts can result in muscle enzyme elevations and potential misinterpretation of results. Encouraging patients to adopt gradual, sustainable exercise routines is often more beneficial than encouraging sudden intensive regimens.

Another important point is the value of reassurance. Abnormal results can provoke unnecessary fear and even lead to further inappropriate testing. By taking a careful history and explaining the benign nature of exercise-induced hyperCKaemia, unnecessary referrals and investigations were avoided.

Finally, this case underscores the importance of communication between patient and doctor. The patient was proactive in seeking help and trusted our practice to interpret his results. By providing clarity, reassurance, and a clear plan, we supported him in continuing his efforts to improve his long-term health without unnecessary alarm.

Case Study 34

Dizziness and Hearing Loss

This 74-year-old woman was seen in Wales in 1978. She lived with her elderly husband in a small bungalow, supported regularly by their daughter. She never smoked, did not drink alcohol, and was a regular churchgoer, attending faithfully with her husband every week.

Her presentation was dominated by dizziness and progressive hearing loss. The story had begun some time earlier when she complained of recurrent dizziness to her GP. Initially this was attributed to ageing, as no clear explanation was found. However, because her symptoms persisted and gradually worsened, she was referred to an ENT surgeon. Despite careful examination, no abnormality was detected. During the same period, she began to develop progressive hearing impairment, again thought to be age-related presbycusis.

A few weeks before hospital admission, she developed pain over the right mastoid region. At first, she managed the pain with simple analgesics, but when it worsened she attended her GP. She was prescribed antibiotics on suspicion of mastoid infection. Unfortunately, there was no improvement, and she was admitted under the acute geriatric team.

Her past medical history included osteoarthritis of the hands, knees, and cervical spine, and hypertension controlled with medication. She had undergone a hysterectomy many years earlier. She walked with the aid of a stick. Her current medications were methyldopa 25 mg twice daily, cinnarizine for dizziness, and co-proxamol for pain. She denied any drug allergies.

On examination, she was pleasant and cooperative, though communication was challenging due to her hearing loss. She was not clinically anaemic and showed no breathlessness. Cardiovascular assessment revealed an irregular pulse at 94 beats per minute, consistent with atrial fibrillation. Blood pressure was 150/82 mmHg. Heart sounds were otherwise normal, with no murmurs, no evidence of cardiac failure, and no peripheral oedema. Respiratory examination was satisfactory, with good expansion and clear air entry.

Neurological examination revealed marked tenderness over the right mastoid. There was no discharge, and otoscopy showed intact tympanic membranes. Significant sensorineural hearing loss was evident. She also displayed nystagmus, a finding that supported vestibular involvement. Importantly, there were no focal neurological deficits, no Babinski reflex, and no features of acute stroke. Her gait, however, was unsteady and unsafe, though she had no other gross neurological abnormalities.

Basic investigations were arranged. ECG confirmed atrial fibrillation. Full blood count showed haemoglobin of 13.5 g/dL with normal indices. ESR was modestly raised. Liver and renal function tests were normal.

Key Questions

1. **What is the differential diagnosis in this case?**
2. **How should this case be managed?**
3. **What is the final diagnosis?**

The differential diagnosis was carefully considered.

Age-related hearing loss (presbycusis) was initially thought to be the explanation, but the fact that her hearing loss was unilateral and progressive argued against this. Presbycusis typically causes bilateral, symmetrical impairment.

Chronic otitis media was another consideration, particularly with mastoid pain, but there was no history of recurrent ear infections, no otorrhoea, and no tympanic membrane abnormalities.

Ménière's disease was also a possibility. It typically presents with vertigo, fluctuating hearing loss, tinnitus, and aural fullness. However, the patient's symptoms were steadily progressive rather than episodic, making this diagnosis less likely.

Vestibular neuritis could cause dizziness and imbalance, but would not explain progressive unilateral hearing loss.

A vascular event such as stroke was excluded, given the absence of focal neurological deficits and the slow progression of her symptoms.

The most concerning possibility was a tumour of the eighth cranial nerve, such as an acoustic neuroma (vestibular schwannoma). The triad of progressive unilateral sensorineural hearing loss, dizziness, and imbalance, combined with mastoid pain and nystagmus, strongly supported this.

At the time, however, diagnostic imaging was limited. CT and MRI were not widely available in local hospitals in the 1970s. Given the seriousness of the suspected diagnosis, referral to a specialist centre was required. After discussion with the consultant, the patient, and her family, a referral was arranged to a tertiary centre in Liverpool.

There, comprehensive investigation confirmed the diagnosis of an acoustic neuroma on the right side. Because of her age and multiple comorbidities, surgical removal was not recommended. Instead, conservative management with supportive care and monitoring was advised. She was transferred back to her local ward for ongoing follow-up and symptom management.

Final Diagnosis

Right-sided acoustic neuroma.

Lesson Learned

This was a challenging and educational case. The patient presented with the triad of dizziness, progressive unilateral hearing loss, and mastoid pain – features which should always raise suspicion of an eighth-nerve tumour such as acoustic neuroma.

The case highlights the importance of persistence in elderly patients with unexplained dizziness. Too often, chronic dizziness in older adults is attributed to 'just ageing.' While ageing can contribute to imbalance, true red-flag features such as unilateral hearing loss and mastoid tenderness should never be dismissed. Careful history and examination are vital.

Another important lesson lies in recognising the limitations of local facilities. In the 1970s, when CT and MRI were not readily accessible, diagnosis required referral to tertiary centres. Even today, when imaging is widely available, this case reminds us of the value of specialist input.

The case also illustrates the importance of progressive symptom review. What began as simple dizziness evolved over time into severe imbalance, significant unilateral hearing loss, and mastoid pain. Each development demanded re-evaluation and reconsideration of the diagnosis.

Finally, it demonstrates the principle of patient-centred care. Although surgical removal of the neuroma might have been considered in a younger patient, in this woman's case her age, comorbidities, and functional status meant conservative management was most appropriate. Supporting her with clear explanations, safety planning, and family involvement was as important as the diagnosis itself.

Case Study 35

Child With Abdominal Rash

This six-year-old girl was seen in 1984, shortly after I had completed my GP training. She was the only child of a professional couple: her father worked as an accountant and her mother as a hospital clerk. The family lived happily in a small bungalow on the outskirts of the city. She had been in good health with no previous medical problems. Her immunisations were up to date, and she had no known allergies.

I was called to see her on a bank holiday. The mother reported that her daughter had developed a rash on the abdomen. I arrived within half an hour. The history was that the child had experienced a mild cough and fever over the previous few days, for which the mother had given paracetamol. The fever seemed to have settled, and the child remained generally well, but the rash had raised concern. The parents denied photophobia, vomiting, or sore throat.

On examination the child appeared comfortable and cheerful. She was examined while standing, and communication was easy. Her neck moved freely with no stiffness. Temperature was 37.6°C, pulse 98 beats per minute. Throat and ears were normal. Heart sounds were normal, chest was clear, and her mental state was normal with no confusion.

Inspection of the abdomen revealed a faint erythematous rash. There were only a few spots, with no blisters, no itching, and no signs of eczema. The rash had developed only within the last 48 hours and was partially blanching.

After completing the examination, I discussed my impression with the parents. In view of the mild temperature, cheerful appearance, absence of meningeal signs, and non-specific rash, my assessment at the time was that this was a viral illness. The parents seemed reassured and accepted this explanation.

Key Questions

1. **What is the differential diagnosis?**
2. **How should this case be managed?**
3. **What is the final diagnosis?**

The most likely impression at first presentation was a viral exanthem. Viral rashes are common in childhood, often associated with a preceding mild fever or respiratory symptoms, and usually self-limiting. Typical causes include enteroviruses, adenoviruses, rubella, and parvovirus B19.

However, the possibility of bacterial meningitis always needs careful consideration when a child presents with fever and rash, even if classical signs are absent. The absence of photophobia, neck stiffness, vomiting, or confusion on this occasion argued against meningitis initially, but these features may appear later, making early recognition difficult.

Other conditions to consider included scarlet fever, which can present with a rash following streptococcal throat infection, though there was no sore throat or 'sandpaper' rash in this case. An allergic rash was also possible, though there was no history of new foods, medications, or exposures.

Another differential is meningococcal septicaemia, which often begins with vague symptoms such as fever and malaise before the appearance of a petechial or purpuric rash. In the earliest stages, the rash can be faint and non-specific, easily mistaken for a viral exanthem. This makes meningococcal disease one of the most dangerous diagnoses to miss.

Kawasaki disease, though rare, should also be borne in mind in children with fever and rash, particularly if features such as conjunctivitis, strawberry tongue, or lymphadenopathy are present. These were not present here, but the condition illustrates how varied rashes in children can be.

In retrospect, the combination of recent fever, new rash, and abnormal cerebrospinal fluid confirmed that meningitis was the underlying cause.

A cautious approach is always required in such situations. A child with a new rash, even if appearing well and without meningeal signs, may still have meningitis or meningococcal disease. The safest course, particularly in primary care, is to refer the child to hospital for observation and further investigation. In hospital, blood tests, cultures, and lumbar puncture would be performed unless contraindicated. Early treatment with intravenous antibiotics is crucial if meningitis is suspected, since delay can have devastating consequences.

For the general practitioner, the challenge is to balance reassurance with vigilance. Many children present with viral rashes and mild illness, but the potentially catastrophic consequences of missed meningitis mean that even small uncertainties should tip the balance toward referral. In this case, the absence of classical features and the child's cheerful appearance made viral illness appear likely. However, with hindsight, referral would have been the safest option.

Three months later a complaint was received, alleging that a diagnosis had been missed. On reviewing my records, I noted the details as above. I later learned that the following day the parents had taken their daughter to hospital because the rash persisted. There she underwent lumbar puncture, which revealed abnormal cerebrospinal fluid with raised cell counts. She was treated empirically for meningitis, recovered, and was eventually discharged. No definite bacterial organism was proven, but she survived and did well.

Final Diagnosis

Meningitis (most likely meningococcal).

Lesson Learned

This case demonstrated that meningitis can present in many different ways. Children may appear relatively well at first, and the rash may be vague and non-specific, yet meningitis should always remain a strong consideration. The absence of classic signs such as photophobia, neck stiffness, and vomiting does not exclude the diagnosis.

The case also highlights the importance of red flags. Any child presenting with fever and rash must be assessed with meningitis in mind. Even when the child looks well, clinicians must keep a high index of suspicion.

Another key lesson is the value of early referral. While hospital observation may appear inconvenient, it provides access to investigations such as lumbar puncture and the immediate initiation of intravenous antibiotics if required. In community practice, where diagnostic tools are limited, observation at home carries risk. When faced with uncertainty, referral is the safest and most defensible option.

This case also carried a medico-legal dimension. The subsequent complaint underscored the professional responsibility to document findings carefully and to communicate clearly with parents about the warning signs of deterioration. Advising parents explicitly to seek immediate hospital care if symptoms change or persist is essential.

Finally, the case was a powerful personal lesson early in my career. It reinforced the need for vigilance, humility, and a willingness to act cautiously in paediatrics. Children with meningitis may initially mimic a mild viral illness. Careful history-taking, close observation, and a low threshold for referral are vital to safeguard the child.

Above all, the message is one of vigilance: when faced with a child with fever and rash, however well they may appear, the possibility of meningitis must never be dismissed.

Case Study 36

Recurrent UTIs

This case was seen in our general practice in the mid-1990s. The patient was a 42-year-old lady, married and living happily with her husband and their four children – three boys and one girl. Her husband was an engineer employed by British Gas, while she was a full-time housewife devoted to caring for her family and running the home. They lived in private accommodation, enjoyed a stable family life, and were well integrated into the community. She had never smoked, did not drink alcohol, and described herself as content and fulfilled in her domestic role. Her health until then had rarely interfered with her family life.

Her medical story went back about a year before she joined our practice. She explained that with her previous GP she had suffered from frequent urinary tract infections. These were diagnosed as cystitis and treated with antibiotics such as trimethoprim and nitrofurantoin. Each time she recovered and thought little more of it. She became accustomed to these attacks and felt confident she could recognise the symptoms herself.

On her third visit to the previous GP, routine investigations were carried out, including a full blood count, liver and kidney function, ESR, and CRP. All appeared normal, apart from two small biochemical abnormalities: calcium was slightly raised, while phosphate was marginally reduced. As she was otherwise well and her infections responded to treatment, these results were filed away and considered of doubtful significance.

Not long afterwards, she experienced an episode of renal colic and was referred to hospital. A CT scan demonstrated a small ureteric stone, which passed spontaneously. She recovered quickly and carried on with her household duties.

Several months later, however, she again developed pain in the renal area, very similar to her previous attack. By this time, she had registered at our practice. She attended one morning and told us in clear terms that she thought she had 'a water infection,' because the pain was identical to her earlier episodes. She was confident in her self-diagnosis, having dealt with several such attacks over the past two years.

We arranged further investigations, repeating calcium, phosphate, renal function, liver function, full blood count, and inflammatory markers. A repeat CT confirmed another small stone in the right ureter. Urine culture grew Escherichia coli, and she was treated with an appropriate antibiotic. The immediate episode settled, but reviewing her history and results together raised concern.

Key Questions

1. **What is your differential diagnosis?**
2. **How do you manage this case?**
3. **What do you think is the final diagnosis?**

Looking back through her previous results, two features stood out: repeated renal stones and persistently raised calcium, accompanied by low phosphate. Even though she had no significant past medical history apart from these events, this biochemical pattern suggested an underlying disorder. She was not on any medication, not even contraceptives, and had no known drug allergies. She had never been treated for endocrine problems, and her family history was unremarkable.

We therefore requested a parathyroid hormone level after discussing the case with an endocrinologist. The result returned unequivocally high, confirming that the biochemical abnormalities were not incidental but explained by parathyroid overactivity. At the endocrinologist's suggestion, an ultrasound of the neck was arranged, which revealed hyperplasia of all four parathyroid glands. This accounted for her persistently raised calcium, reduced phosphate, and recurrent renal stones.

Her care moved largely into the hands of secondary care. She was referred to the endocrinology team, who confirmed the diagnosis and arranged surgery. The first operation involved excision of three-quarters of the parathyroid tissue, leaving a small portion behind. Normally hormone levels fall rapidly within twenty-four hours, but in her case they remained high.

The surgical team concluded that some hyperplastic tissue had been left. Only a week later, before her wound had fully healed, she underwent a second operation. Further tissue was removed, and this time her calcium and phosphate levels began to normalise. Her renal function remained intact, and the recurrent stones ceased.

Although her recovery was prolonged and she endured two operations in quick succession, the outcome was ultimately successful. She returned to her family life without the burden of repeated infections and painful stones. For her, the greatest relief was having a clear explanation for her problems, which had previously been dismissed as 'just another water infection.' It also reassured her husband and children, who had watched her go through repeated episodes of pain and uncertainty without understanding the cause.

Final Diagnosis

Hyperparathyroidism.

Lesson Learned

Small biochemical abnormalities should never be ignored when they fit into a wider clinical pattern. Marginally raised calcium and slightly low phosphate might appear insignificant in isolation, but when paired with recurrent renal stones they should trigger suspicion of parathyroid disease.

Another lesson is that clinicians must not become distracted by frequent urinary tract infections alone, but rather step back and consider what underlying disorder might predispose the patient to repeated events.

This case also illustrates the limits of primary care and the importance of referral to specialists when the picture is unusual. Endocrinologists and surgeons working together provided the definitive diagnosis and cure, but it was recognition of a suspicious biochemical pattern in general practice that set the process in motion.

Finally, the case reminds us of the value of persistence. The patient herself persevered through multiple consultations, and only by revisiting her history in detail were we able to piece together the true explanation. For her, the outcome was not simply medical but personal: she could once again enjoy her family life without fear of further painful and unpredictable attacks.

Case Study 37

Leg Ulcer Above the Ankle

In August 1996, a 38-year-old man presented to the practice with a persistent ulcer on his lower leg.

The patient's social background was important to understand his overall situation. He had been unemployed for several years and was living alone in a council flat. Divorced and without children, he was socially isolated, with little support apart from spending evenings in his local pub. His alcohol intake was heavy, although he denied dependence and said he had never sought help for it. He was not on any prescribed medication and had no known drug allergies. These factors of unemployment, isolation, and alcohol use clearly shaped both his health and his engagement with care.

From the medical point of view, he first noticed a small sore above his left ankle a few weeks before presentation. Believing it to be a minor problem, he treated it himself with over-the-counter creams, but instead of improving, the ulcer gradually enlarged, became increasingly painful, and began to discharge a yellowish exudate. Eventually the discomfort drove him to attend an out-of-hours service, where he was prescribed antibiotics. Despite completing the course, the ulcer failed to heal and continued to worsen.

On presentation at our practice, he appeared alert and cooperative. His general condition was stable: height 180 centimetres, weight 84 kilograms, temperature 37.2°C, pulse 90 beats per minute in sinus rhythm, and blood pressure 145/84 mmHg. Cardiovascular and respiratory systems were normal. There were no clinical features of chronic liver disease such as spider naevi, hepatosplenomegaly, or ascites. Neurological examination was intact, with normal reflexes. In the lower limbs there was no oedema, and peripheral pulses were easily palpable. The ulcer itself was on the medial side of the left ankle, measured about 2 centimetres by 1.5 centimetres, had undermined edges, and contained a purulent yellowish discharge.

Routine investigations were arranged. Blood results showed an elevated mean corpuscular volume (MCV) of 106, consistent with alcohol-related changes, and liver function tests demonstrated a raised gamma-GT and mildly elevated transaminases. Other parameters were within normal limits. A wound swab was negative for bacterial growth. District nurses were engaged to provide regular dressings and ongoing care.

Key Questions

1. **What is your differential diagnosis?**
2. **How would you manage this case?**
3. **What was the final diagnosis?**

Despite these investigations, no definite diagnosis was established. Within the practice, the unusual appearance of the ulcer raised the possibility of pyoderma gangrenosum, and he was referred to dermatology for further assessment. The dermatology team conducted a full review, including a skin biopsy. Histology was non-specific and did not provide a definitive answer.

Nevertheless, the clinical impression supported pyoderma gangrenosum as the most likely explanation, although it remained a diagnosis of exclusion. The recommendation was to continue with conservative wound management using regular dressings, without initiating systemic immunosuppressive therapy.

The differential diagnosis of chronic leg ulcers is broad and must be considered carefully. Venous ulcers are by far the most common, typically occurring around the medial malleolus and often associated with varicose veins, venous insufficiency, and oedema. Arterial ulcers are seen in patients with peripheral vascular disease; they are usually very painful, located on the toes or feet, and associated with diminished or absent distal pulses.

Diabetic ulcers develop on pressure points of the feet and are often complicated by infection and neuropathy. Infective ulcers, both bacterial and fungal, must always be excluded by culture. Less common causes include cutaneous malignancy such as squamous cell carcinoma, vasculitic lesions, and rare inflammatory conditions like pyoderma gangrenosum.

In this patient, the absence of oedema, the presence of intact peripheral pulses, and the lack of diabetes argued against the common causes. Negative culture results excluded infection. The undermined edges, purulent appearance, and failure to respond to antibiotics all pointed towards pyoderma gangrenosum. Although the biopsy was not diagnostic, this remained the most convincing explanation.

Management of leg ulcers depends on the underlying cause. Venous ulcers benefit from compression therapy and sometimes surgical intervention for venous insufficiency. Arterial ulcers require vascular assessment and revascularisation where feasible. Diabetic ulcers demand strict glycaemic control, podiatry care, and infection prevention. Malignant ulcers need excision. Pyoderma gangrenosum, however, usually requires systemic immunosuppression with corticosteroids, ciclosporin, or newer biological agents. In all cases, meticulous wound care and community nursing support are fundamental.

In this man's case, however, the ulcer healed gradually over the course of the following year with conservative management alone. No systemic treatment was given. This outcome surprised both the clinicians and the patient himself, as pyoderma gangrenosum is usually progressive without immunosuppression. Nonetheless, spontaneous healing, although rare, has been described in the literature and represents one of the unusual natural histories of this disease.

Final Diagnosis

Presumed pyoderma gangrenosum presenting as a chronic ulcer on the left ankle.

Lessons Learned

This case highlights several important lessons. First, chronic ulcers require a broad and systematic approach. Clinicians should avoid assuming that all leg ulcers are due to venous insufficiency or infection. Rare conditions such as pyoderma gangrenosum must be considered, particularly when the ulcer does not respond to conventional treatment.

Second, pyoderma gangrenosum is a condition without a definitive diagnostic test. Histology is often non-specific, and the diagnosis rests on exclusion and clinical impression. Multidisciplinary involvement, particularly from dermatology, is vital in such cases.

Third, the case illustrates the impact of social factors on health and disease. The patient's unemployment, isolation, and alcohol use shaped his presentation and complicated his care. Addressing chronic disease often requires a holistic view, taking into account not only the lesion but the wider psychosocial context in which the patient lives.

Finally, the case demonstrates the unpredictability of clinical medicine. Despite diagnostic uncertainty and the absence of specific treatment, the ulcer healed spontaneously. This unusual course serves as a reminder that supportive care and patience may sometimes achieve favourable outcomes, even when aggressive interventions are unavailable or inappropriate.

Case Study 38

Lumps On the Front of Her Lower Legs

This case is unusual in that I must emphasise from the beginning that I did not personally see or examine the patient. The story came to me indirectly. She is the sister of my son's friend, and I only became involved when her brother passed information on to my son, who then sought my advice and my opinion on the matter.

The background goes back about twelve months. This young woman, a school teacher in her mid-twenties, had been feeling generally unwell for about a year. She had no major or dramatic symptoms, but she began to notice lumps developing on the fronts of her lower legs. These were red, raised, uncomfortable, and tender. She promptly consulted her GP. At that stage, the GP reassured her that this might be related to a viral infection. She was prescribed a short course of oral corticosteroids for ten days. The lesions improved but then reappeared about two weeks later, once again on the shins, causing renewed concern.

She returned to her GP, who prescribed another course of steroids. On that occasion, he arranged a plain X-ray and some basic blood tests. Both were reported as normal. At this point, the problem seemed to be recurring without explanation, and the GP concluded that nothing serious was evident, although the patient herself remained anxious.

It was around this time that her brother shared the situation with my son and showed him photographs of his sister's lower limbs. These images came to me, and I felt strongly that the rash represented erythema nodosum. I made it clear, however, that erythema nodosum is not a diagnosis in itself but rather a symptom of an underlying disorder. I insisted that her brother convey this to her, and that further investigation was required to find the cause.

I asked a number of screening questions, even though the information was second-hand. I inquired about cough, night sweats, weight loss, family history of chronic disease, diarrhoea, blood in the stools, and any current or past medications. All of these were denied. She did not smoke, she did not drink alcohol, and she was not taking any regular treatment, including contraceptive pills. Apart from common coughs and colds, she had never suffered significant illness. Socially she was content, living happily with her family and leading a professional, stable life with no evident stressors or risks.

At this stage, before revealing the eventual outcome, it is appropriate to pause for reflection.

Key Questions

1. **What is your differential diagnosis of the problem?**
2. **What investigations would you arrange in order to establish the underlying cause?**
3. **What is the final outcome or the diagnosis?**

I emphasised once more to the family that erythema nodosum is not a disease but only a symptom. The causes are many, and sometimes no definite cause is found, in which case it may be attributed to a self-limiting viral infection. More often, however, there is a specific trigger. Common causes which must be considered include streptococcal throat infection, sarcoidosis, tuberculosis, and inflammatory bowel disease, among others. The list is long, but these are the most important conditions to bear in mind.

Investigations must be directed toward uncovering one of these causes. I asked the family to return to her GP and to request further evaluation, particularly a chest X-ray. Unfortunately, this request was declined, because she had already had a plain X-ray which had been reported as normal. Dissatisfied with this outcome, the family took matters further and arranged a private consultation, where a repeat chest X-ray was performed. This time the film revealed clear evidence of pulmonary tuberculosis. From that point, the whole case changed direction and required urgent referral to a specialist clinic.

The final diagnosis was erythema nodosum secondary to pulmonary tuberculosis. Once this was confirmed, appropriate referral and treatment followed. She was seen in a specialist chest clinic, commenced on standard anti-tuberculous therapy, and her case was notified to the public health authorities, as required by law.

Lesson Learned

This case illustrates how erythema nodosum must always be regarded as a symptom, never as a diagnosis. It is a cutaneous marker of underlying disease, and the clinician's task is to search carefully for the cause. Sometimes the condition is due to a self-limiting viral illness, but often there is a serious underlying disorder that requires treatment. Sarcoidosis, streptococcal throat infection, tuberculosis, and inflammatory bowel disease are among the most important associations to keep in mind.

The psychological impact on the patient must not be underestimated. In this case the young woman was distressed to discover that her condition had been missed for many months and that she had been repeatedly reassured without the underlying cause being found. Counselling and support were essential to help her cope with the diagnosis and the temporary interruption to her work, and reassurance was needed to maintain her confidence in the medical process.

Finally, the public health implications of tuberculosis are significant. As a school teacher, she was in daily contact with children and colleagues.

Notification to the health authorities and contact tracing were essential, both to protect her family and to safeguard the wider community. The role of the chest clinic is not only to treat the patient but also to ensure that those at risk are identified and, where necessary, protected with prophylactic therapy.

The key message is clear: ERYTHEMA NODOSUM IS NOT A DISEASE, BUT A SIGNAL. It requires persistence, thorough investigation, and awareness of the broader medical, psychological, and social consequences once the underlying cause is uncovered.

Case Study 39

Urethral Discharge

This case occurred during my trainee year, within the first two months of starting general practice, when I had very little experience and was still learning the realities of day-to-day practice. It proved to be an interesting dilemma and, in many ways, a challenge.

The patient was a 37-year-old man, employed as a car mechanic. He smoked around 30 cigarettes a day. He was married with one child, lived with his family in his own private home, and enjoyed a fairly ordinary social life.

He presented with a complaint of urethral discharge, which he described as creamy in colour. The discharge was associated with pain on passing urine. Apart from this, he reported no other symptoms. He was especially worried about the appearance of the discharge. When asked about his sexual history, he strongly denied any sexual contact outside of his marriage. He insisted he had never had relations with anyone other than his wife since marrying, and he was firm about this, and repeated it several times.

His past medical history included mild asthma, for which he used a beta-agonist inhaler occasionally, especially during the summer pollen season. The asthma never really troubled him significantly. He was not known to have any allergies. He drank alcohol only on social occasions when out with his wife. He was not on any regular medication apart from his inhaler.

On examination he was slim and appeared well. He measured 182 centimetres in height and weighed 77 kilograms. His blood pressure was 137/81 mmHg, temperature a little over 37°C, and his pulse 88 beats per minute in sinus rhythm. Systematic examination of the cardiovascular, respiratory, neurological, and abdominal systems was all normal.

I explained to him that, at this stage, it was difficult to identify the problem with certainty. I therefore took a urethral swab and sent it to the pathology laboratory for testing. Three days later the results came back, and the swab confirmed gonococcal infection.

When I informed him of this result, he immediately denied it. He became angry and agitated, saying it was impossible. He doubted the diagnosis, insisted that I was wrong, and began to question my competence. I explained clearly that the result was not my opinion but the official report from the pathology laboratory. I told him it was my responsibility to explain the findings and arrange management, not to blame him. I offered to contact the laboratory myself and speak to them about the result. After this, he went silent.

The next day he returned, this time with his wife. I then discovered that she had visited the practice three or four days earlier, complaining of what she thought was cystitis. She had been seen by another partner and treated empirically, without a urine culture being sent. From her manner during our consultation, I strongly suspected she was the source of the infection. She avoided eye contact, looked down, and remained completely silent. She never offered a word of explanation or defence.

Despite my attempt to explain, both husband and wife dismissed what I told them. They left the consultation and then asked the receptionist about me. They questioned whether I was truly a doctor, asked who had given me a licence to practise, and told the receptionist I knew nothing. In short, they insulted me behind my back. At that time, as a young trainee, it was not easy to hear, but I chose to ignore it outwardly.

What is your action plan in this case?

At that stage, I was not sure of the right course of action. I admitted to myself that I lacked experience and felt uncertain. I turned to my trainer, the senior partner in the practice, for advice. He told me to ignore the personal insults, as they were a reaction to the stigma of the diagnosis.

He reminded me that my duty was not to argue with the patient but to ensure proper management. His advice was to refer the patient directly to the genitourinary medicine clinic. The GUM clinic could then take responsibility for treatment, partner notification, and contact tracing. In his view, that was the safest and most appropriate course of action.

Lesson Learned

This case was a valuable lesson early in my career. It taught me that sometimes the biggest challenge is not making the diagnosis but dealing with the patient's reaction to it. Denial, anger, and attempts to shift blame are common when the diagnosis carries social or moral stigma. It is the doctor's responsibility to remain calm, objective, and professional, even in the face of hostility.

It also reinforced the importance of clear communication. The doctor must make it absolutely clear that the diagnosis is based on laboratory evidence, not on personal judgement. The role of the GP is to manage the problem with compassion and professionalism, not to accuse or condemn.

Most importantly, I learned that when faced with a confirmed diagnosis of gonococcal infection, the correct course of action is referral to the genitourinary clinic. These clinics are best equipped to carry out contact tracing, offer appropriate treatment, and provide counselling in a confidential environment. The GP must recognise their responsibility, but also know when to hand over to specialist services.

Finally, this case reminded me of the need for resilience. As a young doctor, it was difficult to be insulted and undermined, but I had to learn that such comments should not distract me from my duty. Professionalism means focusing on what is right for the patient and the wider public health, even when the patient resists or denies the truth.

The key message is clear: GONOCOCCAL INFECTION DEMANDS A CALM, PROFESSIONAL RESPONSE AND APPROPRIATE REFERRAL, EVEN IN THE FACE OF DENIAL OR ANGER.

Case Study 40

Mid-Thoracic Pain

This case took place in 1973, during my earliest days as a young doctor. I had only recently graduated from medical school and was rotating between orthopaedics and surgery. With very limited experience, I encountered a patient whose condition left a permanent mark on my memory.

The patient was a 35-year-old shopkeeper, married with three children. He was a quiet and religious man who did not smoke or drink alcohol. His family life was stable, and he spent most of his time either at work or with his wife and children. The only physical strain in his life came from occasional heavy lifting while carrying goods in his shop.

He first noticed a dull, constant pain in the middle of his back, roughly in the region of the dorsal vertebrae D8 to D10. At the time, he dismissed it as the result of lifting too much. He rested for a few days, but the pain did not settle. Instead, it persisted and gradually worsened, interfering with his ability to continue his daily work.

There were no constitutional symptoms. He did not have fever, night sweats, or weight loss. The pain did not radiate. His appetite remained normal, and he had no morning stiffness. His bladder and bowel functions were perfectly intact, and he experienced no weakness or numbness in his limbs.

His past medical history was unremarkable, aside from the usual childhood illnesses such as coughs, colds, and occasional dysentery, all of which had resolved without complication. He did report an allergy to sulfonamide drugs, still in common use at the time, and was taking indomethacin for pain relief.

At first, he sought help locally. Several doctors – including general practitioners and even an orthopaedic surgeon – saw him. One injection of an anti-inflammatory drug gave only temporary relief, and the pain returned almost immediately. His condition continued to worsen, forcing him to seek further attention.

When examined at the local hospital, he appeared slim, about 180 centimetres in height and weighing 72 kilograms. His pulse, blood pressure, heart, and lungs were normal. Abdominal examination was unremarkable. Neurological assessment of the limbs was also normal at this stage. The only finding was tenderness over the mid-thoracic spine.

Investigations were limited. A plain radiograph of the thoracic spine showed lytic destruction of the vertebral bodies of D8 and D9, with possible early involvement of D10. No paraspinal calcification was seen. Blood tests were normal, except for an ESR of 50 mm/hour. This suggested inflammation, but did not point to a clear cause. On the presumption of infection, the patient was given a two-week course of antibiotics, which brought no improvement. With no CT or MRI available, the local team could do no more.

Recognising the seriousness of the situation, and with partial support from his government, the patient travelled to the United Kingdom to seek specialist help. This was a major step for him and his family, but it reflected the desperation of his situation.

When he arrived in the UK, he was seen privately by an orthopaedic team. He still appeared otherwise well, slim and in no distress except for his persistent mid-thoracic pain. Yet now, something new had developed. Examination revealed spasticity in both lower limbs. Reflexes were brisk, and plantar responses were up-going. These upper motor neurone signs indicated compression of the spinal cord.

Further investigations were undertaken. Repeat radiographs confirmed the destructive lesion. Myelography, then the best available test, showed indentation of the cord. The impression was of a destructive vertebral process threatening paralysis if not relieved.

He was counselled extensively. The surgeons explained that surgery was essential if he was to avoid paraplegia, but they also warned him of the risks. Paralysis was a real possibility, and even if successful, recurrence was common. Despite the risks, surgery was the only option.

He underwent decompression and debridement of the diseased vertebrae. The operation was technically demanding, as the surgeons were aware that rupture of any cystic structure could spread the disease. With meticulous care, the cord was decompressed.

Post-operatively, he improved partially. Importantly, he did not lose bladder or bowel function, and he avoided complete paraplegia. His pain was eased, but spasticity and some functional limitations remained. He eventually returned home with residual disability but enough independence to manage daily life.

Key Questions

1. **What is the differential diagnosis of this case?**
2. **What is the final diagnosis?**

The differential diagnosis included several possibilities. Tuberculosis of the spine - Pott's disease - was common in his part of the world and had to be strongly considered. Pyogenic infection and brucellosis were other infective causes. Parasitic disease, especially hydatid disease, though rare in the spine, was possible, particularly given his background. Amoebic abscesses were well known in the tropics but were rarely found in bone. Neoplastic causes also needed to be considered, such as vertebral haemangioma, primary bone tumours, or secondary deposits from thyroid, renal, breast, or lung malignancies.

Ultimately, the diagnosis was established at surgery. The lesion was a hydatid cyst of the spine involving D8 and D9, encroaching upon the spinal canal and causing cord compression. It was an unusual and extraordinary presentation, far more familiar to physicians dealing with cysts of the liver or lungs.

For me, as a young doctor, the case was unforgettable. It underlined the importance of considering geography and travel history when faced with an unusual clinical picture. It reminded me that persistent, destructive back pain must not be dismissed, especially when neurological signs emerge. It demonstrated how formidable hydatid disease can be in the spine, where cysts infiltrate bone, are difficult to remove completely, and tend to recur.

In the 1970s, without MRI or CT, diagnosis was almost impossible before surgery. Even today, spinal hydatidosis remains a challenging disease, but in this man's case, the outcome was not without merit. He retained sphincter control, he avoided paraplegia, and though he lived with disability, he returned home still able to care for himself and his family.

The final diagnosis was hydatid cyst of the spine, affecting D8 and D9, with compression of the thoracic cord.

Lesson Learned

Persistent and destructive back pain should always prompt thorough consideration of serious underlying causes. In regions where tuberculosis or hydatid disease is endemic, these must be kept firmly in mind. The appearance of neurological signs such as spasticity, brisk reflexes, and up-going plantar responses are red flags for cord compression and demand urgent intervention. Spinal hydatid disease is particularly difficult to treat because of its infiltrative nature, the risk of intra-operative rupture, and its high recurrence rate. Even today, management remains complex, but the preservation of neurological function should remain the central goal.

Case Study 41

Sudden High Temperature and Vomiting in a 12-Year-Old Child

This case I encountered in 1974 in Libya, during a short period of work there. At that time, I was responsible for a village with a population of around six to seven thousand people. The nearest hospital was about 30 kilometres away, and transport was extremely limited. Cars were few, drivers not always available, and arranging any transfer took considerable time and difficulty.

The patient was a 12-year-old boy who lived happily with his parents and sister. His family were tidy, kind, and helpful, living a modest but content life on a small farm. The boy was cheerful, attended school regularly, and was well integrated in the village community. He had no history of serious illness and had grown up as a healthy child.

One morning, the boy suddenly woke with a very high and persistent fever. He was unable to lift his head from the pillow, and his condition alarmed his family. There was no diarrhoea, no cough, no runny nose, and no rash of any kind. The main accompanying symptoms were repeated vomiting and a severe headache. His parents were particularly worried about how rapidly his illness had come on and how unwell he appeared.

His past medical history was unremarkable, apart from occasional coughs and colds from which he had always recovered well. He had no known allergies and was not on any regular medication. He was brought promptly to the medical centre – the only facility available in the village, where I was working as the sole doctor.

On general examination, he was clearly ill and could not communicate well. He struggled even to respond to simple questions. His temperature was 39°C, with a pulse of 95 beats per minute, and he was not sweating.

Systematic examination revealed no noticeable rash at any point. His neck was checked carefully several times, but there was no stiffness to suggest meningitis. His throat was not inflamed, his ears were normal, and there was no discharge. His chest was clear, with the trachea central, respiratory rate 16, and no added sounds. Cardiovascular examination revealed normal heart sounds with no murmurs. His abdomen was soft, with no palpable liver or spleen and no tenderness. His limbs showed no abnormalities.

Key Questions

1. **What is the likely diagnosis?**
2. **What would you do in such a situation, in a remote place with limited facilities?**
3. **What is the final diagnosis?**

This was a remote village with no access to routine laboratory testing. Sending blood cultures or swabs was not practically possible, and transport to the hospital was long and difficult. In such situations, one has to rely heavily on clinical judgment, local knowledge, and the epidemiology of disease in the area. Balancing all these factors, the most likely diagnosis was typhoid fever. I therefore commenced empirical treatment immediately. An injection of chloramphenicol was given, followed by Buscopan to control vomiting, and oral chloramphenicol was then continued.

The boy was admitted to the centre overnight for observation. Despite treatment, his fever remained high and he was still unable to lift his head. The next day, I visited him at home. He looked no better. His pulse was racing and irregular, almost certainly due to the persistent fever. His father became increasingly anxious about his son's deteriorating state. By this point, about 40 hours into treatment, I decided the safest option was transfer to hospital. An ambulance was requested, though it took some time to arrive.

Before transfer, I reflected on the important differential diagnoses. Viral infection was possible, but there were no respiratory signs, no rash, and no clear viral features. Other bacterial infections could not be entirely ruled out, but there was no evidence in the chest, ears, or urinary system to support this. A broad infective process remained possible, but the epidemiology of the region and the boy's presentation strongly pointed towards typhoid fever.

The hospital was run by Yugoslavian staff, who did not speak English, but through an interpreter I was able to explain the clinical picture, the local epidemiology, and the treatment already administered. We left the boy there around midnight. The next morning, his father and I returned. To our great relief, we found him in the hospital yard, walking, cheerful, whistling, and completely transformed.

The hospital staff agreed that the most likely diagnosis was typhoid fever. A Widal test was performed, which later returned positive. A blood culture was attempted, but it was not surprising that nothing grew, as antibiotics had already been given. His blood count showed leukopenia, which fitted the picture of enteric fever. He was kept in hospital for a short time before being discharged, with instructions for review if necessary.

The pattern of his recovery was entirely consistent with the known action of chloramphenicol, which typically takes about 48 hours to show effect. This explained why he had remained acutely ill for nearly two days, but then suddenly improved. Looking back, the clinical diagnosis of typhoid fever was strongly supported by epidemiology, examination, and eventual serology. In a resource-limited setting, reliance on clinical skills and careful monitoring proved essential.

Final Diagnosis

Typhoid fever.

Lesson Learned

The important lesson from this case is the need always to take account of local epidemiology when practising in remote areas, since the pattern of disease there may differ greatly from that in more developed settings. In such circumstances, empirical treatment is often the only realistic option, because transport is difficult, laboratories are distant, and cultures or serology are not readily available.

Chloramphenicol remains effective in the treatment of typhoid fever, but it often takes up to 48 hours before significant clinical improvement is seen, which means that patience, careful monitoring, and close observation are essential. Whenever there is no improvement, or if deterioration occurs, transfer to hospital should be arranged, even if distances and logistics make this difficult. Finally, good communication with families is vital. In situations where resources are limited, keeping relatives informed and involved helps to maintain trust and reassurance during a difficult time.

Case Study 42

High Temperature for a Few Weeks

Awareness of the local epidemiology is essential. It guides the clinician toward the most likely diagnosis when laboratory support is absent. Another important point is hygiene. Typhoid fever spreads by faecal-oral contamination, and public health measures to improve sanitation remain central to preventing the disease. In remote areas, where facilities are limited, these principles become even more important.

This case I saw overseas in 1974 in Libya, where I served for a couple of months near the border between Libya and Tunisia. The area was thinly populated, but there was a small medical centre with a nurse working alongside me. The clinic was situated directly by the Mediterranean sea, in a beautiful and peaceful setting. On average, I would see about ten to 15 patients a day.

One day a very pleasant gentleman came to see me. He was 31 years old, married with two young children, and worked at the border checkpoint. He lived about 20 kilometres away and had his own car, so he had no problem travelling.

He complained of severe headache and feeling feverish for about a week. During this time, he had lost his appetite and had been rather constipated. He denied cough, diarrhoea, vomiting, or rash. Overall, he described feeling generally unwell. He had tried over-the-counter remedies, including paracetamol and indomethacin, which reduced the fever temporarily but never for long. After seven days of persisting symptoms, he became concerned and came to the clinic.

His past medical history was unremarkable. He denied any allergies and took no regular medication.

On examination, he was a tall man, measuring 184 centimetres in height and weighing about 75 kilograms. He looked well nourished and did not appear anaemic or short of breath, but he was visibly worried, particularly as a young man with two small children. His blood pressure was 130/80 mmHg, pulse 75 beats per minute, and temperature 38.9°C. Interestingly, although his temperature was high, his pulse remained relatively low, varying between 80 and 90 beats per minute.

Cardiovascular examination revealed normal heart sounds without murmurs. His chest was clear: trachea central, vesicular breath sounds bilaterally, and no added sounds. Abdominal examination revealed no scars or tenderness. The liver was not palpable, but I thought I could just feel the tip of the spleen, though I could not be entirely confident. His central nervous system examination, including careful checking for neck stiffness, was normal. Throat and nasal passages were clear, and both upper and lower limbs were entirely normal.

Key Questions

1. **What do you think might be wrong with this patient?**
2. **How would you manage the case in such a setting?**
3. **What is the final diagnosis?**

This was again a remote area with no laboratory facilities nearby. The closest pathology and serology services were at least 70 miles away. In such circumstances, clinical judgment and an understanding of the local epidemiology are crucial. Common diseases in that part of Libya at the time included contagious conditions such as diphtheria, malaria, typhoid fever, and pyogenic infections. Less common but possible differentials included

Hodgkin lymphoma and urinary tract infections, but there were no findings to support those.

Given the clinical picture, the constipation, the fever, and the possible palpable spleen, the most likely diagnosis was typhoid fever. I prescribed chloramphenicol from the clinic's supply, to be taken four times daily for at least two weeks, and advised him to return after three days for review, knowing that chloramphenicol often requires at least 48 hours to show full effect. The gentleman agreed to this plan, and I explained to him that in my opinion the most likely diagnosis was typhoid fever.

He did not return after three days and was effectively lost to follow-up. About a month later, however, he reappeared at the clinic. He greeted me warmly, sat down, and explained what had happened. He had travelled to Tripoli, quite a long distance from our village, where he underwent further investigations. To cut the story short, the diagnosis of typhoid fever was confirmed. He had told the doctors there that I had already started him on chloramphenicol, and they advised him to continue the same medication. He completed the course and made a full recovery.

Final Diagnosis

Typhoid fever.

Lesson Learned

This case, together with the 12-year-old boy I described earlier, illustrates how typhoid fever can present in different ways, in different ages, but in similar epidemiological settings. One was a child with acute severe illness, the other an adult with persistent fever, headache, and constipation. Both were seen in rural Libya, and in both, the diagnosis rested heavily on awareness of the local pattern of disease. The important lesson is that typhoid fever can present in many guises: sometimes with diarrhoea, sometimes with blood in the stool, sometimes with skin rash, and at other times with constipation and fever. It may strike in different age groups and wear a different clinical 'coat,' but the underlying disease is the same.

This case, when read alongside Case 41, highlights the contrast between a child and an adult presenting with the same illness under similar circumstances. Such comparisons strengthen the point that a single disease can manifest in very different ways, and the clinician must always remain alert to these variations.

Awareness of the local epidemiology is essential. It guides the clinician toward the most likely diagnosis when laboratory support is absent. Another important point is hygiene. Typhoid fever spreads by faecal-oral contamination, and public health measures to improve sanitation remain central to preventing the disease. In remote areas, where facilities are limited, these principles become more significant.

Case Study 43

Haematemesis

This case took place in 1973 during my second hospital rotation as a newly-qualified doctor. I was working as a house officer on a busy medical ward. Only a few months into my first year of practice, it was during this time that we encountered a patient who presented as an emergency with a dramatic and worrying condition.

The patient was a 45-year-old man who was brought to hospital late at night after suddenly vomiting a large amount of altered blood. The vomit was described by his relative as a black, tarry substance rather than bright red blood, suggesting the bleeding had been present long enough for partial digestion to occur. Much of the initial history was given by his relative, as the patient himself was weak and tired on arrival.

The patient had apparently previously been in good health, with no history of indigestion, no known episode of melaena, and no prior abdominal complaints. He had never noticed pain radiating to the back or any other relevant symptoms. His illness appeared to begin abruptly on the evening of admission when he started vomiting black material persistently. Alarmed, his family carried him to hospital, travelling from outside the city to reach us.

His past medical history was essentially nil, as far as could be established. He had never suffered from any serious illnesses and had not been under medical care for any chronic condition. He was not taking any regular medication and had no known drug allergies. Socially, he was a smoker of around 20 cigarettes per day, but denied heavy alcohol consumption.

On arrival at the ward, the patient appeared slightly pale, but was not sweating profusely and did not seem to be in significant pain. He weighed approximately 70 kilograms and was 177 centimetres tall. His temperature was normal. His blood pressure was 110/70 mmHg with a pulse rate of 100 beats per minute - slightly rapid but regular. His breathing was not distressed.

Examination revealed no palpable abdominal tenderness and no signs of ascites. However, the liver was felt about two fingerbreadths below the costal margin; it was smooth in outline and non-tender. Both upper and lower limbs were unremarkable, and the neurological examination was grossly normal, apart from the evidence of vomitus. There were no other immediate alarming findings.

Initial investigations were quickly performed. His haemoglobin was low at 8.9 g/dL, confirming significant blood loss. The white cell count was mildly raised at 12,000. Kidney function tests were within normal limits, and liver function tests were intact and unremarkable.

Immediate priority was resuscitation and stabilization. The patient was kept nil by mouth, and intravenous infusions were commenced. A blood transfusion was urgently required, but in those days the system was far less sophisticated than today. A recall person was sent to arrange cross-matching, and he was found to be group B. Donors from outside the hospital were waiting at the gate to provide blood. They were paid around £2 per pint. A pint was taken from one donor, then another, and transfused directly into the patient, with additional units stored in the ward refrigerator.

Alongside transfusion, gastric suction was applied using the standard apparatus, which in those days was often used both therapeutically and to reduce the risk of aspiration pneumonia. Electrolytes, particularly potassium, were monitored closely during resuscitation. The patient was given intravenous fluids, mainly normal saline, while blood replacement continued.

Despite these measures, the bleeding seemed to continue, as evidenced by ongoing aspiration of altered blood from the stomach. At that time, however, our therapeutic options were severely limited. There were no proton pump inhibitors and no H2 receptor blockers, such as cimetidine or ranitidine, and endoscopy was not available in that hospital. The approach was essentially supportive - blood replacement, gastric suction, and close observation - in the hope that gastric bleeding would settle spontaneously.

Key Questions

1. **How would you manage this case, apart from what has already been described?**
2. **What is your differential diagnosis?**
3. **What do you think was the final diagnosis?**

The differential diagnosis was, in reality, limited to a few possibilities: gastric ulcer, duodenal ulcer, gastric carcinoma, oesophageal varices, and less commonly a bleeding disorder from a haematological disease. Without endoscopy, it was impossible to be certain, and the clinical features could fit more than one of these possibilities.

In practice, the gentleman continued to bleed. Every time I aspirated the stomach, the suction returned black fluid. I felt increasingly anxious. The senior physician was at home and in any case, there was little more he could offer under the circumstances. I struggled through the night on my own.

Eventually, I turned to the resources available on the ward. There was a copy of Harrison's Principles of Internal Medicine, the American reference book. I searched through it, looking for guidance on how to stop upper gastrointestinal bleeding. One suggestion caught my attention: the instillation of very cold water, close to zero degrees Celsius, into the stomach, holding it for ten to 15 minutes, then aspirating and repeating.

With no other options available, I decided to try this method. After two cycles of cold water lavage, the aspirate cleared. Instead of black, turbid material, the suction began returning clear fluid. I was both surprised and relieved. The bleeding had apparently stopped. I remained on the ward until 2 am to be certain and reassured myself that no further bleeding had occurred.

The stomach remained free of blood. The senior physician reviewed him the next morning, agreed that the bleeding had stopped, and advised us simply to continue supportive care. The patient was kept in the ward for three more days. His haemoglobin rose steadily after repeated transfusions, and by the fourth day he was sitting in the chair beside his bed, smiling and talking to his relative. He was discharged home soon afterwards, fully recovered.

The final diagnosis, based on the clinical picture and reasoning, was that the bleeding had been due to portal hypertension, most likely secondary to schistosomiasis (bilharziasis), a common disease in that part of the world.

Lesson Learned

This case was unique for me, not only because of the dramatic nature of the upper gastrointestinal bleed, but also because of the limitations of medical practice in 1973. There was no endoscopy to identify the source, no proton pump inhibitors, no H2 blockers, and very little in the way of definite drug treatment. In such an environment, doctors were forced to improvise with whatever resources they had. Cold water gastric lavage may seem primitive by modern standards, and many doctors today have never heard of it. Yet, on that night, the bleeding stopped, and the patient survived.

The experience taught me that sometimes in medicine, especially in resource-limited settings, resourcefulness and determination can make all the difference. It also reminded me how challenging and isolating medical practice can feel when technology and drugs are lacking, and responsibility falls squarely on the shoulders of the doctor at the bedside.

Case Study 44

Mental Problems with Breast Carcinoma

This patient was a 75-year-old lady who was admitted to a psychiatric hospital. She was a widow with two grown-up daughters who visited her regularly. She had never smoked, did not drink alcohol, and lived peacefully and happily at home.

While I was working in psychiatry, she was admitted because of mental health issues. Her history stretched back about twelve months. She had begun to experience auditory hallucinations, claiming that she could hear God speaking to her. She was firmly convinced of this and would argue about it with her daughters. Eventually, they persuaded her to see her GP.

At the GP consultation, she presented as sensible, fully oriented, with intact memory and good judgment. There were no disturbances of smell, and her central nervous system examination showed no localised signs - no weakness, no brisk reflexes, no fasciculations, and normal limb movements. The GP tried to convince her to take medication or attend further clinics, but she was adamant that there was nothing wrong with her, explaining that she only conversed with God intermittently and took instructions from Him.

Her background history included hypertension, for which she was taking methyldopa with good control. She also had carcinoma of the left breast. A lump had been identified, but given her age and her refusal of surgery, the matter was left. There was no ulceration or local lymph node involvement.

Despite her daughters' efforts, she initially refused further psychiatric assessment. Eventually, however, she agreed to be admitted to hospital, and this was when I first encountered her. On admission, her history was essentially the same as that recorded by the GP. She reported no sleep disturbance, continued to cook for herself, and remained independent in daily living.

On examination, she looked well, with no shortness of breath and good peripheral perfusion. Her pulse was 84 beats per minute in sinus rhythm and her blood pressure was 150/79 mmHg. Heart sounds were normal, chest clear, and abdominal examination showed no organomegaly or tenderness. Neurological examination was unremarkable. The breast lump was about 4 cm × 5 cm with no ulceration, peau d'orange, or axillary nodes.

The patient's mental state remained stable, apart from the encapsulated delusion: she believed God was speaking to her and discussing many issues with her. She was stubborn, sometimes arrogant, and difficult to interview, but with persistence we managed to obtain adequate information. For about two weeks she refused all medication, but eventually agreed to start antipsychotics.

After around three weeks of treatment, the patient began to complain of constipation, abdominal pain, and difficulty passing stool. Her abdomen felt tight, and she was clearly uncomfortable. At this stage I was still a relatively junior doctor, and I asked the senior registrar to review her. He examined her and wrote in his report that he could not find anything significant.

Key Questions

1. **How would you evaluate this case further?**
2. **What do you think was the final diagnosis?**

Basic investigations, including full blood count, renal and liver function tests, vitamin B12, and folate, were all unremarkable. Despite this, her constipation and abdominal discomfort persisted. Considering the uncertainty, we sought a surgical opinion from the nearby hospital.

On rectal examination, the surgeon identified a rectal stricture with narrowing of the lumen. The conclusion was that her carcinoma of the breast had metastasised to the rectum, producing this stricture. This was an unusual and striking finding, as metastasis to the rectum from breast cancer is relatively rare.

The patient therefore had multiple coexisting problems: a psychiatric condition with delusional belief and auditory hallucinations; carcinoma of the breast, untreated and now metastatic; and constipation and abdominal pain due to rectal stricture secondary to metastasis.

Final Diagnosis

Breast carcinoma with rectal metastasis causing stricture, alongside late-onset psychosis.

Comment

This case highlights the complexity of managing elderly patients with both psychiatric and physical illnesses. The psychiatric problem was characterised by a fixed paranoia, also known as an encapsulated delusion. Patients in this situation can appear otherwise normal, but it is impossible to convince them against their belief. This creates particular difficulty in deciding whether to respect autonomy or to enforce treatment under the Mental Health Act.

At the same time, her physical complaints could not be overlooked. The abdominal pain and constipation turned out to be the result of a rectal stricture due to metastasis from breast cancer. This unusual spread of disease shows the importance of linking problems together rather than treating them as separate diagnoses. Constipation and rectal narrowing were not isolated problems - they were directly related to her breast cancer.

The senior registrar initially failed to identify the abdominal cause, underlining the importance of involving colleagues from other specialties. It was the surgeon's examination and experience which revealed the true diagnosis. This reminds us that multidisciplinary collaboration is essential when patients present with complex, overlapping issues.

Respecting patient autonomy is another key theme. While her psychiatric condition raised the possibility of compulsory admission, her independence in daily life and the absence of risk to herself or others meant that her autonomy needed to be respected. Balancing autonomy with medical responsibility is particularly important in elderly patients facing multiple health challenges.

Lessons Learned

This case demonstrates several important principles. Fixed paranoia, or encapsulated delusion, is a psychiatric condition where patients may appear otherwise normal but remain unshakably convinced of their belief, making treatment decisions challenging. Respecting patient autonomy is critical, even when compulsory admission is considered, and this must always be balanced with safety and clinical judgment.

Another lesson is the importance of linking pathologies, rather than treating problems in isolation: here, constipation and rectal narrowing were directly linked to breast cancer metastasis. Finally, the case highlights the value of interdisciplinary collaboration, as psychiatry alone could not provide the full answer: surgical expertise was required to uncover the underlying diagnosis.

Case Study 45

Right Shoulder Pain

This case was seen in 1983 during my GP training year. The patient was a 60-year-old retired foundry worker. He was married, living with his wife in a semi-detached house in the suburbs of the city. A regular churchgoer, he attended services two or three times a week, including Sundays, accompanied by his wife. They had two daughters living locally who visited occasionally, but the couple generally managed independently and did not require much help.

He initially presented to his GP with pain in the right shoulder. The pain began gradually, described as a dull ache, especially on lifting the arm. He self-medicated with paracetamol, which provided only partial relief. Over the following weeks the pain worsened, prompting him to return to his GP. On examination there was only a slight limitation of movement, which was interpreted as a frozen shoulder. He was prescribed co-proxamol, a popular analgesic at the time, but the pain continued and became more troubling.

A follow-up consultation was arranged, during which the GP requested an X-ray of the shoulder. As part of the view, the upper lung fields were included. The report noted fibrosis in the apex of the lung, which the radiologist interpreted as an old scar from previous tuberculosis. The GP filed this as a past abnormality of no current concern.

During this period the patient noticed loss of appetite and weight loss of around three kilograms. He also complained of low energy, contrasting with his previous active lifestyle of gardening, walking, and attending church. Dissatisfied with his care, he changed practice and joined the surgery where I was training.

At his first consultation in our practice he was seen by a colleague, who prescribed stronger anti-inflammatory medication for the presumed frozen shoulder. I then saw him at his second visit.

Taking a full history, I explored his appetite, weight, bowel habits, cough, fever, and other systemic symptoms. He denied diarrhoea, vomiting, chest pain, or fever, but confirmed poor appetite, weight loss, and low energy.

His past medical history included diverticulitis, for which he occasionally used laxatives, and appendicitis in childhood. He also had a history of chronic cough and wheezing, managed with inhalers, and had smoked 20 cigarettes a day for many years, although he had stopped ten years earlier. He was taking Adalat 10 mg three times daily for hypertension. He drank only a couple of pints of beer weekly.

On examination, he showed signs of weight loss but was not clinically anaemic. There was no shortness of breath at rest. Temperature was 36.5°C, pulse 100 beats per minute in sinus rhythm, and blood pressure 115/78 mmHg. Cardiovascular examination was normal. Chest examination revealed the trachea centrally placed, with scattered wheezes and crepitations consistent with chronic smoking. There was early finger clubbing. The right apex was difficult to assess clearly. There was no pleural effusion.

Abdominal examination showed no organomegaly or tenderness. The locomotor system showed symmetrical limbs with normal reflexes. Apart from the right shoulder discomfort, there were no musculoskeletal abnormalities. Urinalysis was clear, with no protein, leucocytes, or blood.

Key Questions

1. **What is the differential diagnosis?**
2. **How would you manage this case?**
3. **What do you think was the final diagnosis?**

At this point the differential diagnosis included frozen shoulder, osteoarthritis of the shoulder joint, referred pain from lung or rib pathology, osteoporosis with possible rib fracture, and rarer causes such as brachial plexus neuritis.

I reviewed the patient's notes and found the previous radiology report, which had described the apical fibrosis as an old TB scar. Since I had not seen the original film myself, I arranged for a repeat chest X-ray.

Further investigations included full blood count, ESR, CRP, liver and renal function tests. The haemoglobin was 10.9 g/dL, showing mild normocytic anaemia. ESR was elevated at 61 mm/h, and CRP was 45 mg/L. Liver and renal function were within normal limits.

The repeat chest X-ray, when compared to the earlier report, showed progression of the apical shadow, extending more widely into the upper lung. This explained his shoulder pain and weight loss. In the context of his smoking history and finger clubbing, carcinoma of the lung was now the most likely diagnosis, rather than old TB scarring.

The patient was urgently referred to the chest clinic. Within two weeks, bronchoscopy and biopsy confirmed carcinoma of the lung.

This diagnosis was devastating for the patient and his family. His shoulder pain, initially thought to be musculoskeletal, had in fact been a presenting feature of apical lung cancer. Unfortunately, despite referral, his disease progressed rapidly, and he died within two months of diagnosis. His wife required considerable support and counselling following his death.

Final Diagnosis

Carcinoma of the lung presenting with shoulder pain.

Comment

This case highlights the dangers of misinterpretation. The radiological finding of apical shadow was labelled as an old TB scar without correlation to the clinical picture. The patient's persistent pain, weight loss, and smoking history should have prompted further review earlier.

Shoulder pain can sometimes be a misleading presentation of thoracic disease. In this case it reflected direct extension of an apical tumour, rather than a primary musculoskeletal disorder.

This case also illustrates the importance of revisiting a diagnosis when symptoms do not improve with treatment. Symptomatic management alone can mask serious underlying disease if the root cause is not sought.

Lesson Learned

If symptoms do not improve with treatment, the diagnosis must always be re-examined. Persistent pain, weight loss, or systemic features should trigger renewed investigation. Radiological findings must be considered in conjunction with the clinical picture; apical fibrosis in a smoker should raise the suspicion of carcinoma, not simply be dismissed as old tuberculosis.

This case underlines the importance of correlating clinical history, risk factors, and imaging together. Lung cancer may present deceptively, and early recognition can change the outcome.

Case Study 46

Seizures in a 28-Year-Old

In 1980, whilst I was working in general medicine, a 28-year-old woman was admitted to the medical ward through the Accident and Emergency department. She had suffered a fit at her workplace.

The patient had been working in a residential home for the past four years. She was married, living happily with her husband, a taxi driver, and their nine-year-old daughter. They owned their own home and described their life as contented.

When she presented to casualty, she was stabilised with intravenous diazepam. Once recovered, she gave a history of feeling generally unwell for the past three months. She described tiredness, sluggishness, and loss of energy, which contrasted with her usual dynamic and active lifestyle. She had also lost three kilograms in weight. She denied cough, diarrhoea, vomiting, chest pain, abdominal pain, or urinary symptoms, although she had been experiencing occasional low-grade fever.

She had already seen her GP before this admission. Blood tests at that time showed a haemoglobin of 11 g/dL, indicating mild normocytic anaemia, and an ESR of 27 mm/h. Chest X-ray was normal. Clinical examination at the time had not revealed any significant abnormality.

Over the weeks leading up to admission, the patient continued to feel unwell. Nursing staff at her workplace recorded episodes of fever, which she treated herself with paracetamol. Then, without warning, she suffered a fit at work. Colleagues restrained her and called an ambulance.

On arrival to the medical ward, following stabilisation, she appeared not clinically anaemic. Her pulse was 100 beats per minute, blood pressure

130/82 mmHg, temperature 37.8°C. Cardiovascular and respiratory examinations were normal. The trachea was central, with vesicular breath sounds and no added sounds. Abdominal examination showed a liver palpable three fingerbreadths below the costal margin, but the spleen was not palpable.

Neurological examination revealed mild weakness of the right leg, particularly in the extensor muscles, with brisk reflexes and an up-going plantar response. The other limbs were normal. There was no cranial nerve abnormality, no double vision, and no squint. Neck stiffness was equivocal but not definitely positive.

Baseline investigations included full blood count, ESR, renal and liver function tests, and C-reactive protein. Her ESR was 35 mm/h, slightly raised. Other investigations were within normal limits.

During admission, she suffered further seizures, some associated with transient loss of hearing. At this point, the possibility of an intracranial lesion was strongly suspected. Given the fever, weight loss, and neurological deficit, the differential included brain tumour, cerebral abscess, or parasitic cysts.

Key Questions

1. **How would you evaluate this case further?**
2. **What do you think was the final diagnosis?**

At that time, CT scanning facilities were limited. After discussion with my consultant, we referred her urgently to the regional neurosurgical centre. Given the localised neurological signs, neurosurgical assessment was considered essential.

The neurosurgical team proceeded to exploratory surgery. On opening the skull, they found and evacuated a cystic abscess. Samples were sent for culture and sensitivity. Final microbiology confirmed Mycobacterium tuberculosis.

Final Diagnosis

Tuberculous cerebral abscess.

Comment

This case illustrates how tuberculosis can present in unexpected and severe forms. The patient, originally from Mauritius in East Africa and living in the UK for ten years, had no chest involvement on X-ray, yet developed a cerebral abscess due to tuberculosis. Her presentation with seizures, fever, and subtle neurological signs was the first indication of the disease.

The diagnosis required persistence and referral to a tertiary centre. Without neurosurgical exploration, the cause would not have been identified. This highlights the importance of recognising that tuberculosis can affect any organ system - not only the lungs, but also bone, lymph nodes, or, as here, the brain.

Another important aspect is the role of collaboration. The medical team recognised the limits of local investigation and sought neurosurgical input promptly. Once the abscess was drained and identified as tuberculous, further management was transferred to the tuberculosis clinic for initiation of anti-tuberculous therapy.

Lesson Learned

This case emphasises several important lessons. Tuberculosis remains a wide-ranging and dangerous disease, capable of affecting any part of the body, including the central nervous system. A normal chest X-ray does not exclude tuberculosis. Clinicians should always keep a high index of suspicion when faced with unexplained fever, weight loss, raised ESR, and focal neurological signs.

Equally important is the role of tertiary services. In this case, neurosurgical intervention was decisive both for treatment and for establishing the diagnosis. Finally, tuberculosis is not just an individual problem but a public health concern. Contact tracing and community protection are essential once a diagnosis is confirmed.

Case Study 47

Pregnant Lady with Weakness, Loss of Weight

In the winter of 1981, while working in the Department of General Medicine, I received a call from my consultant late in the afternoon. He requested that I attend the obstetric ward to review a patient who had been admitted directly from the outpatient clinic. After completing my blood pressure clinic, at around 4.30 pm, I walked to the ward. It was a typical winter day - cold, damp, and windy.

The patient was a 24-year-old woman of Asian origin who had immigrated to the UK at the age of ten with her family, settling in the suburbs of the city. She was in her second pregnancy at 32 weeks' gestation, with one healthy four-year-old child at home. She lived happily with her husband in private accommodation and had a large extended family in the local area. She had never smoked, did not drink alcohol, and had no known allergies.

The patient reported that she had been feeling generally unwell for several weeks, with fatigue and weight loss. Her past history was significant for childhood asthma, poorly controlled, requiring frequent courses of oral corticosteroids. At the time she was using both steroid and beta-agonist inhalers.

Of particular note, she had returned to the UK ten weeks earlier after an extended visit to her original home in Pakistan. While abroad, she had experienced two episodes of frank haematuria. She had undergone investigations at a local hospital, but no cause was found and her symptoms resolved spontaneously. She denied diarrhoea, vomiting, cough, or systemic symptoms, and there was no family or personal history of tuberculosis.

On examination, she appeared somewhat tired, but not overtly anaemic. Her weight was 68 kilograms and her height 166 centimetres. Her temperature was 37.6°C, pulse 96 beats per minute, blood pressure 110 mmHg systolic, and respiratory rate 18 per minute. Chest examination revealed vesicular breath sounds with scattered expiratory wheezes but no crepitations or effusion. Peak expiratory flow was 450 L/min, which was satisfactory.

Cardiovascular examination was unremarkable. Neurological examination showed no neck stiffness or focal deficits. Abdominal examination revealed a gravid uterus consistent with 32 weeks' gestation but no hepatosplenomegaly or masses.

Initial investigations included a full blood count, ESR, renal and liver function, G6PD screen, and urine analysis with culture. Results showed haemoglobin 10 g/dL with MCV 78 fL, ESR 37 mm/h, and normal renal and liver function tests. Urinalysis demonstrated proteinuria (2+) with around 10 red blood cells per high-power field (normal 0-2). The initial urine culture was sterile.

Key Questions

1. **Given these findings - fever, anaemia, raised ESR, and sterile pyuria with proteinuria - what is your differential diagnosis?**
2. **What would be your next step in the management of this patient?**
3. **What do you think was the final diagnosis?**

Given these findings – fever, anaemia, raised ESR, and sterile pyuria – the possibility of glomerular disease or interstitial nephritis was considered. I discussed the case with my consultant, who agreed further evaluation was necessary. A urologist was consulted, but given the negative culture, they felt their input was limited. Repeat urine cultures and a chest X-ray were arranged, along with immunological tests including ANA and rheumatoid factor, all of which returned negative. The chest X-ray showed no abnormality. Abdominal ultrasound also showed no significant findings.

Differential diagnoses at this stage included pyelonephritis, renal carcinoma (such as hypernephroma), or renal calculi, but these did not fully explain the sterile pyuria and persistent proteinuria. Despite repeated cultures, the patient's low-grade fever persisted (38.0-38.1°C) with ongoing fatigue and anaemia. Her ESR later rose to 60 mm/h.

At this point, I revisited the patient's history, noting two important factors: her recent stay in a tuberculosis-endemic country, and her immunocompromised state from repeated corticosteroid use. With a high index of suspicion, I requested specialised testing for urinary tuberculosis. Subsequent culture confirmed the presence of Mycobacterium tuberculosis, sensitive to standard anti-tuberculous therapy.

Final Diagnosis

Urinary tuberculosis during pregnancy.

Comment

This case illustrates the critical importance of recognising sterile pyuria with haematuria in a patient returning from an endemic region. A thorough history is invaluable, particularly regarding recent travel to high-risk areas. Red flags such as unexplained fever, persistent sterile pyuria, proteinuria, and raised ESR should always prompt consideration of tuberculosis, even when routine cultures are negative.

Repeated urine cultures and specialised testing eventually revealed the rare pathogen – Mycobacterium tuberculosis. The patient's asthma and frequent corticosteroid use had likely weakened her immune system, increasing susceptibility. The fact that the patient was pregnant meant that additional multidisciplinary care was required to ensure the best possible outcome for both mother and child.

Lesson Learned

This case is a valuable reminder of the diagnostic challenges posed by atypical presentations of tuberculosis. It highlights the importance of persistence in the face of unexplained fever, weight loss, and urinary abnormalities. Careful history-taking, attention to travel history, and awareness of immunosuppression are key to identifying unusual but important causes such as urinary tuberculosis.

Case Study 48

Five-Year-Old Boy with Pain in the Genital Area

This case took place in 1996 during a particularly cold winter. I had been working an out-of-hours shift and was just finishing when the controller asked if I could attend one final call. Although I was at the end of my shift, I agreed to go.

The patient was a five-year-old boy who had been reviewed by his GP earlier that morning, approximately 18 hours previously, with pain in the genital area. The GP had examined him, reassured the parents that there was nothing of major concern, and advised paracetamol with instructions to call back if problems continued.

When I arrived at the house, the boy's mother gave me a clear account. Her son was an otherwise healthy child, with no significant past medical history apart from dry skin, which was controlled with moisturisers. He was fully immunised, had no known allergies, and had been well until this sudden episode. She explained that his pain had started suddenly in the right testicle, worsening over the past 24 hours. Despite paracetamol and ibuprofen, he had been unable to sleep due to the severity of the pain.

On examination, the boy was visibly distressed but afebrile, with a temperature of 37.1°C. No rashes or spots were present. The right testicle was markedly tender, rock-hard, and warm, though not visibly red. There were no systemic signs of infection. His heart rate was 100 per minute, and the remainder of the clinical examination was normal.

At this stage, I immediately recognised the urgency of the presentation.

Key Questions

1. **What might be wrong with this child, and what is the differential diagnosis?**
2. **How would you manage this case?**
3. **What do you think was the final diagnosis?**

I explained to the mother, in plain language, that her son needed to be taken to hospital without delay. Initially she wished to wait until the morning, but I stressed that any delay could cause permanent damage, including the loss of the testicle. She then agreed to immediate transfer.

I called an ambulance with blue lights and contacted the on-call paediatric surgical registrar at the children's hospital, emphasising the seriousness of the case. Fortunately, the ambulance arrived quickly and transported the child.

The following morning, I telephoned the hospital to follow up. Sadly, I learned that the testicle was gangrenous and had to be removed. The delay between the initial consultation and his hospital admission had proved fatal for the organ.

The differential diagnoses at presentation included testicular torsion, strangulated inguinal hernia, and acute epididymo-orchitis, although the last is uncommon at this age. The final diagnosis was testicular torsion with gangrene, leading to orchidectomy.

Some weeks later I was summoned to court as a witness after the parents lodged a complaint against their GP, alleging negligence. Having worked previously as a police surgeon, I was familiar with giving evidence, but nevertheless found the process demanding.

On the day of the hearing, I received the case documents and prepared myself carefully. Standing in the witness box, I was confronted by the full weight of legal procedure. The prosecution barrister pressed me with rapid and often repetitive questions, probing for any inconsistency. The defence barrister followed with equal intensity, seeking clarification and reassurance about the standard of care. Each question required clear, measured replies; there was no room for speculation or casual remark.

The atmosphere was tense. Although the case did not revolve around my actions, I still felt the pressure of being under scrutiny. The formality of the court, the stern expressions of the jury, and the adversarial tone of the barristers made the experience exhausting. By the end of the day, I was mentally and emotionally drained. It was a stark reminder that medicine does not exist in isolation from the legal system; clinical decisions are often later dissected in a courtroom, far removed from the urgency of the bedside.

Two weeks later, I was informed that no concerns had been raised about my involvement. My actions had been judged appropriate and timely. Unfortunately, my GP colleague was referred to the GMC in London, and I later learned that the family was awarded £35,000 in compensation.

Lesson Learned

This case reinforced the reality that acute scrotal pain in children must always be regarded as testicular torsion until proven otherwise. It is one of the few true surgical emergencies in paediatrics, where every hour makes a difference between salvage and loss. Other diagnoses, such as acute epididymo-orchitis or a strangulated inguinal hernia, can present in a similar fashion, but they must never delay urgent surgical exploration.

Equally important was the lesson in communication. Parents may not always grasp the seriousness of the situation, particularly when the child does not appear gravely unwell. It requires calm but firm explanation, in simple non-medical terms, to convey the urgency and ensure compliance with immediate referral. In this case, had I not insisted on transfer, the outcome might have been even worse.

The legal aftermath offered further lessons. A missed or delayed torsion not only devastates the child and family but also exposes clinicians to complaints, GMC proceedings, and compensation claims. Even when one's own conduct is beyond criticism, being drawn into the legal process is stressful and draining. Court appearances are emotionally taxing, and doctors can feel vulnerable under the intensity of cross-examination. This underlines the importance of precise documentation and decisive action, which remain the strongest protection for any clinician.

For younger doctors, this story highlights that medicine involves not just science and compassion, but also accountability. Every clinical encounter has the potential to be scrutinised in retrospect, sometimes years later, in a legal forum. Recognising this early in one's career helps to instil habits of careful note-keeping, unambiguous communication, and prompt referral when doubt exists.

Above all, this experience was a powerful reminder that the welfare of the child comes first. Swift recognition, prompt referral, and effective communication with parents are essential - not only to preserve health and function but also to safeguard the clinician from professional and legal negative consequences.

Case Study 49

Shortness of Breath

This case occurred in 1996 and involved a colleague of ours, a general practitioner who had been registered with our practice since 1990. For reasons of confidentiality I shall refer to him as DB. He was 59 years old, a highly-regarded partner in a neighbouring local practice, and a well-known figure within the medical community.

DB was a cheerful and pleasant gentleman, married to a medical secretary. They had two grown-up children who lived locally and remained closely involved in family life, visiting their parents regularly. He never smoked and consumed only three to four pints of beer a week. He and his wife lived in their own comfortable home, enjoying what appeared to be a happy and stable marriage.

Professionally, DB was a dynamic figure. I encountered him often at health authority meetings, which I frequently chaired, and I also met him in my capacity as a GP colleague at least once a week. He was energetic, engaged, and well-respected.

One afternoon, following a quarterly health authority meeting, he asked if we might have a private word. I suggested that he come to my surgery the next morning. During that consultation he confided in me that he had been losing weight over the preceding few weeks, amounting to a full stone. His appetite was waning, and he noticed breathlessness with even minimal exertion. He denied cough, diarrhoea, vomiting, or other obvious symptoms.

DB's past medical history included allergic sinusitis, episodes of low blood pressure, and gastro-oesophageal reflux disease. Otherwise, he had been relatively healthy, with no known history of liver disease, no alcohol excess, and no other major comorbidities.

On examination he appeared unusually tired and looked unwell. He was clearly short of breath, though not tachypnoeic at rest. His temperature was 36.9°C. The trachea was central. Chest examination revealed no obvious crackles or wheeze. His abdomen revealed the liver edge palpable three centimetres below the costal margin. It was smooth and non-tender, though I could feel a firm fullness in the right lobe, suggesting underlying pathology. His cardiovascular and neurological examinations were within normal limits.

Key Questions

1. **What differential diagnoses should be considered in this patient?**
2. **How would you manage it?**
3. **What ultimately was the final diagnosis?**

Given the severity of his symptoms and the unexplained weight loss, I arranged an urgent set of blood tests: full blood count, liver function tests, urea and electrolytes, C-reactive protein, ESR, and serum proteins.

The next day the results returned. His liver enzymes were significantly abnormal, with both transaminases and alkaline phosphatase more than double the upper limit of normal. CRP was 37 and ESR 56 mm/hour, suggesting significant inflammation. Renal function was preserved.

I contacted DB immediately and explained that these findings required urgent secondary care input. He agreed and was referred without delay to the regional hepatology team.

Differential Diagnosis

At this stage several possibilities were considered. The most likely was a malignancy, given the weight loss, anorexia, and declining health. A primary hepatocellular carcinoma or metastatic carcinoma to the liver were both possible. Other considerations included lymphoma, especially given the systemic symptoms, or an underlying chronic infection such as tuberculosis. Though less likely, poisoning or toxic exposure was also considered. Stress alone could not explain the biochemical abnormalities. The pattern of liver enzyme derangement, however, strongly suggested an intrahepatic pathology, making hepatoma the leading differential.

Within a week DB attended hepatology outpatients. Before his appointment, he telephoned to say that his abdomen had become rapidly distended and that both ankles were swollen. I advised him to proceed directly with his planned appointment. At the clinic, the consultant was sufficiently concerned to admit him immediately.

During admission, further investigations were performed. His liver function tests deteriorated further. Alpha-fetoprotein was markedly elevated, pointing towards a malignant process. An abdominal ultrasound revealed a large mass within the liver. A biopsy, carried out under imaging guidance, confirmed the diagnosis of hepatocellular carcinoma (hepatoma).

Tragically, DB's condition declined rapidly. Despite supportive measures, he died shortly afterwards in hospital.

Lesson Learned

This was an especially painful case, not only because of the clinical outcome but also because the patient was a professional colleague and friend. It illustrated starkly how aggressive primary liver cancer can be. DB had presented with relatively non-specific symptoms – weight loss, loss of appetite, and exertional breathlessness – and within a matter of weeks he was dead.

In general practice, unexplained weight loss is always a red flag. Although common causes include gastrointestinal or haematological malignancies, one must also consider hepatoma, especially in patients with abnormal liver function tests. Even in the absence of a background of cirrhosis or alcohol misuse, hepatocellular carcinoma can strike, and it often presents late with vague, insidious symptoms.

Another important lesson lies in the relationship between doctors and their own health. DB, being a GP, recognised that something was wrong but delayed formal investigation until he felt compelled to confide in me. Doctors frequently minimise their own symptoms or assume they can self-manage, sometimes to their detriment. This case is a reminder that doctors are not immune to illness and should seek timely medical care when unwell.

The case also demonstrated the importance of rapid referral. As soon as the abnormal liver function results were available, urgent hepatology involvement was essential. Unfortunately, even with prompt action, the disease was already too advanced to allow meaningful intervention.

For teaching purposes, the pattern of liver enzyme abnormalities is also important. A predominant rise in alkaline phosphatase, accompanied by raised transaminases, often points to an obstructive or infiltrative process within the liver, including malignancy. Recognising such patterns at the earliest stage can guide the GP to expedite investigations and referral, even before more specific markers such as alpha-fetoprotein are obtained.

Emotionally, caring for a colleague is always difficult. Delivering news to a fellow GP carries a different weight, as one is speaking to someone who fully understands the implications of each investigation and result. The professional boundaries blur with personal connections, making the experience more intense.

Finally, this case highlights the need for vigilance in evaluating non-specific symptoms. Weight loss, fatigue, and subtle changes in wellbeing may herald serious disease. As general practitioners we are often the first to detect these signals, and our role is pivotal in initiating timely investigations.

Above all, the story of DB underscores how fleeting health can be, even for those who dedicate their lives to caring for others. It is a sobering reminder of the vulnerability of patients and doctors alike, and of the responsibility we carry in remaining alert to the silent signs of serious illness.

Case Study 50

Lower Limbs Swelling

This case was not from my practice, but one I came across during my postgraduate medical training. In 1979, while attending a clinical meeting, one of the physicians presented it. I found it interesting and memorable, and I felt it was worth including in this book because of the important clinical lessons it illustrates.

The patient was a 55-year-old man, originally from Lancashire, who had been referred by his GP for investigation of lower limb swelling. He had previously spent ten years working for an oil company in Egypt, residing in a Swiss-managed city during that time. His main complaint was swelling of both legs, which had first appeared a few months earlier. The swelling became most noticeable in the evening and tended to improve by the following morning. Apart from this, he felt generally well, but the symptom worried him enough to seek medical attention.

On further enquiry, he recalled two previous episodes of haematuria during his years in Egypt. These episodes had been investigated in Cairo. No definite cause was found, but bilharzia (schistosomiasis) was suspected, and he was treated for it. He had not experienced haematuria since then. His past medical history was otherwise unremarkable, with no history of chest pain, renal disease, or recurrent urinary infections apart from those episodes. He was a non-smoker and took no regular medications.

On clinical assessment he appeared confident, articulate, and in no distress. He did not look anaemic. His height was 178 centimetres and weight 80 kilograms. His pulse was 80 beats per minute, regular, and his blood pressure was 135/78 mmHg. Cardiac examination was unremarkable.

The respiratory system was normal, with central trachea, vesicular breath sounds, no added sounds, and good chest expansion. There was no clubbing.

Abdominal examination revealed no clinical signs of ascites. The liver edge was palpable 3 centimetres below the costal margin, smooth and non-tender. The spleen was just palpable. There were no spider naevi, no palmar erythema, and no cutaneous stigmata of chronic liver disease. Neurological examination was normal, with no motor or sensory deficits and reflexes intact.

Key Questions

1. **What do you think the differential diagnosis in this case?**
2. **How would you proceed in this case?**
3. **What is the final diagnosis?**

The differential diagnosis for bilateral lower limb swelling in this context included renal disease such as nephrotic syndrome, though there was no proteinuria or urinary abnormality. Chronic liver disease with portal hypertension, possibly secondary to bilharzia or cirrhosis, was a strong consideration. Venous obstruction was possible, though there were no clinical findings to support this. Cardiac failure was also a possibility, but there was no history or evidence of ischemic heart disease, cardiomyopathy, or heart failure clinically.

Routine investigations were requested: full blood count, ESR, renal and liver function tests, hepatitis B serology, and urine analysis. The results showed haemoglobin of 11 g/dL with MCV of 107, indicating macrocytic anaemia. Liver enzymes were mildly elevated, and bilirubin was slightly raised.

Renal function, including sodium, potassium and urea, was within the normal range. These findings raised strong suspicion of alcohol-related liver disease despite the patient's claim of modest alcohol intake. Further tests included vitamin B12 and folate, which were within the normal range. Gamma-glutamyl transferase (GGT) was markedly elevated – about five times the upper limit of normal.

When confronted with these results, the patient initially repeated his story of modest drinking. However, with more careful and persistent questioning, he eventually admitted to a different history. He had in fact been dismissed from two jobs because of alcohol-related issues, confirming significant alcohol misuse. The final diagnosis was alcohol-induced liver cirrhosis with portal hypertension.

This was an important case because the initial history suggested bilharzia-induced liver disease, which is indeed common in Egypt and can lead to portal hypertension and cirrhosis. However, the laboratory results pointed strongly towards alcoholic liver disease. Only after sensitive but firm re-questioning did the patient disclose his true level of alcohol consumption. It illustrates how denial and minimisation are frequent when patients are questioned about alcohol intake. What they describe as 'just a couple of pints a day' may, when explored further, amount to very heavy consumption over weekends or in social settings.

Lesson Learned

History-taking must be thorough and persistent. Patients often underreport alcohol consumption, so careful, detailed questioning is essential. Biochemical evidence should never be ignored; an elevated MCV together with a markedly raised GGT are strong markers of excess alcohol intake and should always prompt the clinician to revisit the history. Social context must also be taken into account. Living overseas, working in isolated environments, or spending long periods at sea may predispose individuals to heavy alcohol use, and this should remain in mind when assessing such patients.

Case Study 51

Exertional Shortness of Breath in a 14-Year-Old Girl

While practising as a general practitioner, I encountered a 14-year-old girl from Yemen who presented with central cyanosis. She had travelled from a remote area of Yemen to visit her sister in the United Kingdom. She was accompanied by her mother and was registered at the practice, as she was staying for more than three months. During her new patient check-up, I immediately noticed striking cyanosis, which prompted further enquiry.

Her mother explained that the girl had appeared like this for quite a number of years, with persistent blueness most obvious around her nose, and that she also suffered from exertional shortness of breath. She had been seen by a local doctor in Yemen on several occasions and had received unspecified medication without significant improvement. Despite her symptoms, she attended school and managed to function reasonably well.

Her birth history was uncomplicated, born at 37 weeks. According to her mother, she had received all routine immunisations, though no documentation was available. She reported no allergies and was not taking regular medication.

On examination, she was not breathless at rest, but obvious central cyanosis was present together with digital clubbing. Her pulse rate was 80 beats per minute, temperature 36.9°C. I heard a loud systolic murmur at the right sternal edge. There were no signs of heart failure such as raised jugular venous pressure or peripheral oedema. Her respiratory system was unremarkable: trachea central, vesicular breath sounds, no added sounds. She was mentally alert, communicated normally, and her neurological examination was grossly normal with no neck stiffness or limb abnormality.

Key Questions

1. What is your differential diagnosis?
2. How do you manage this case?
3. What is the final diagnosis?

The differential diagnosis in this case centred on two main considerations. The first was cyanotic congenital heart disease, which includes a recognised group of five classic conditions, though it is unnecessary to list them all here as that is not the purpose of this book. The second was Eisenmenger syndrome, in which a long-standing left-to-right shunt, as seen in ventricular septal defect, atrial septal defect, or patent ductus arteriosus, eventually reverses to a right-to-left shunt due to rising pulmonary pressures, thereby producing central cyanosis.

As I was working in primary care and had experience in cardiology after spending twelve months in a cardiology department before becoming a GP, I recognised the need for urgent referral. I arranged for her to be seen in a cardiac clinic, and the consultant agreed to review her within two weeks.

Six weeks later, we received a detailed communication from the hospital cardiologist. The patient had undergone echocardiography, ECG, chest X-ray, and routine blood tests including renal function and haemoglobin. These confirmed the diagnosis of a congenital cardiac arteriovenous malformation, specifically a patent ductus arteriosus. Three months later the consultant surgeon informed us that she had undergone successful surgical correction of the malformation. At follow-up, she appeared dramatically improved: her cyanosis had resolved and she reported feeling far more energetic.

This case illustrated a congenital arteriovenous communication that had failed to close after birth. Initially, the shunt was from left to right, but with progressive pulmonary hypertension the pressure gradient reversed, producing a right-to-left shunt and resulting in hypoxia and central cyanosis. If untreated, this would eventually have led to heart failure and severe complications.

Final Diagnosis

Patent ductus arteriosus.

Lesson Learned

This case underscores the profound impact of vigilant clinical observation in diagnosing serious conditions, even in seemingly routine settings. The presentation was subtle in one sense - the patient appeared well enough to attend school - but central cyanosis and clubbing combined with a systolic murmur were unmistakable clues to an underlying congenital heart defect. Prompt referral to a specialist centre enabled life-saving surgical intervention. The case highlights the value of careful observation, the need never to ignore central cyanosis, and the importance of considering congenital causes in young patients.

Central cyanosis should always prompt investigation, no matter how well the patient appears. It also reminds us that patients from areas with limited healthcare access may harbour undiagnosed conditions into adolescence. Finally, it reinforces the role of the GP as a gatekeeper: recognising the abnormal, initiating referral, and ensuring timely management that can transform a patient's life.

Author Biography

Dr Omar J Hassouna

General Practitioner, Medical Author, Former Chair of Local GPs

With nearly five decades of experience working within the National Health Service (NHS), Dr Hassouna has devoted his professional life to clinical medicine, medical leadership, and education. His medical career began in London in 1976 with a clinical attachment, after which he undertook a wide range of hospital posts that laid the foundation for a broad and practical understanding of medicine.

Diverse Medical Experience

Dr Hassouna's early hospital work included paediatrics, geriatric acute medicine in Wales, and psychiatry, where he developed a strong appreciation of mental health conditions such as anxiety, depression, and psychosis. As a medical registrar, he gained further experience in diabetes, haematology, respiratory medicine, cardiology, and gastroenterology, managing both acute and chronic medical conditions. He also spent time in gynaecology and obstetrics, further widening my clinical exposure and reinforcing the importance of holistic patient care.

These formative years shaped his diagnostic thinking and clinical judgement, skills that later became central themes in his medical writing.

Transition to General Practice

In 1983, Dr Hassouna transitioned into general practice, initially joining a training practice before becoming a partner in 1984. This move required a significant shift from hospital-based medicine to managing undifferentiated presentations in the community. Over time, he established and led several dedicated clinics, including antenatal, postnatal, hypertension, diabetes, respiratory (COPD and asthma), thyroid, and gout clinics. These services enabled comprehensive and continuity-based care tailored to community needs.

He also established a WHO-recognised Travel Clinic, providing risk assessment, travel advice, vaccinations including yellow fever, and official certification. This service supported both local patients and travellers from further afield.

Leadership and Administrative Roles

From 2007 to 2010, Dr Hassouna served as Chair of the local GPs. During this period, he attended monthly Primary Care Trust (PCT) meetings and chaired numerous GP forums. This role provided first-hand insight into the interface between frontline general practice and healthcare policy. It strengthened his understanding of system pressures, governance, and the practical challenges faced by clinicians working within evolving NHS structures.

Out-of-Hours and Urgent Care Experience

Throughout the 1980s and 1990s, Dr Hassouna worked extensively in out-of-hours services. This was an era before mobile phones, electronic records, or centralised triage systems, often requiring long journeys and rapid decision-making under difficult conditions. These experiences were instrumental in developing clinical resilience, independence, and pragmatic problem-solving skills.

Following 2000, he also worked within Urgent Care Centres, adapting to newer models of emergency and unscheduled care and witnessing first-hand the increasing pressures on acute services.

Forensic and Social Medicine

Alongside general practice, Dr Hassouna served as a Police Surgeon, working closely with law enforcement on cases involving drug misuse, assault, sexual offences, and deaths in custody. This role demanded meticulous clinical assessment, legal awareness, and close collaboration with police and courts.

He also worked with social services, assessing patients for disability and mobility allowances. Conducting home visits provided invaluable insight into the social determinants of health and reinforced the importance of contextual medicine beyond clinical settings.

Continuing Professional Development

Dr Hassouna remains committed to lifelong learning, obtaining postgraduate diplomas in Dermatology (Cardiff University) and Diabetes Care (Warwick University). These qualifications strengthened his specialist input within primary care and informed both his clinical and educational work.

Qualifications

MBCHB, Baghdad
LMSSA, London
Practical Dermatology Diploma, Cardiff University
Diploma in Diabetes Care, Warwick University

Authorship and Educational Contribution

Drawing on decades of real-world clinical experience, the author has published three medical books, each with a distinct but complementary focus:

Challenging Scenarios in Medicine (2025)

This book presents complex and often high-risk clinical situations encountered in general practice, accident and emergency departments, hospital wards, and community settings. It focuses on safe decision-making, uncertainty, and practical management in challenging circumstances.

Real-World Challenges in Clinical Medicine (2026)

Building on the first book, this volume places greater emphasis on everyday clinical dilemmas faced by GPs and junior doctors, particularly in under-resourced and time-pressured environments. It highlights diagnostic pitfalls, communication challenges, premature discharges, and situations where clinicians are left managing risk with limited support.

Practical Approaches to Clinical Diagnosis (2026)

This book adopts a topic-based, structured approach to diagnosis. It is designed to help clinicians reach accurate diagnoses efficiently by focusing on common presentations, pattern recognition, and clinically relevant reasoning. The aim is to save time, reduce unnecessary investigations, control costs, and enhance patient safety.

Together, these books reflect a progression from complex scenarios, to real-world pressures, to practical diagnostic frameworks.

A note from the Author

Over the decades, I have witnessed profound changes in the NHS, particularly since 2005. Increasing workload, workforce shortages, population growth, ageing demographics, resource limitations, and administrative inefficiencies have placed the system under sustained strain. Staff morale has declined, and patient presentations have become more complex. These realities provided strong motivation for translating clinical experience into educational resources for the next generation of clinicians.

My professional journey reflects a sustained commitment to patient care, medical education, and mentorship. Through my clinical work, leadership roles, and writing, I aim to support medical students, junior doctors, and general practitioners in navigating the increasing complexity of modern medicine and maintaining high standards of safe, thoughtful clinical practice.

Dr Omar Hassouna